Breaking Thru
the Fibro Fog

Scientific Proof
Fibromyalgia is Real!

Kevin P. White, M.D., Ph.D.

With a foreword by Dr. I. Jon Russell

Wortley Road Books

www.wortleyroadbooks.com

Breaking Thru the Fibro Fog™ - Scientific Proof Fibromyalgia Is Real
Copyright © 2010 by Kevin Patrick White, M.D., Ph.D.

Publisher: Wortley Road Books, 343 Dundas Street, #302, London Ontario N6B 1V5
www.wortleyroadbooks.com

Printed in Canada

National Library of Canada Cataloguing in Publication Data

Breaking Thru the Fibro Fog™ - Scientific Proof Fibromyalgia Is Real
White, Dr. Kevin P.
ISBN number: 978-0-9867881-0-9

A percentage of proceeds from every sale will go to the American Fibromyalgia Syndrome Association (AFSA) in support of fibromyalgia research, advocacy and education.

Cover design by Darlene Steele
www.divinedynamicdesigns.com
dsteele@divinedynamicdesigns.com

How many ears must one man have

before he can hear people cry?

Blowin' in the Wind

Bob Dylan

ENDORSEMENTS OF
Breaking thru the Fibro Fog

"God Bless You, Dr. White!"

Ardith Heller (fibromyalgia sufferer)

"BRAVO!!!!!! and there is a lot of clapping going on. For all Fibromyalgia patients, families, physicians, lawyers and researchers, this is a Proverbial Masterpiece. I feel that this book "Breaking Thru the Fibro Fog" is an antidote in itself. BRAVO!"

D. Steele (author, and fibromyalgia sufferer)

"Dr White is an excellent advocate for fibromyalgia and to be commended for this excellent, thorough book to help patients with pain and other debilitating symptoms of fibromyalgia."

Janice Sumpton (pharmacist, fibromyalgia sufferer and support group leader)

"This book presents, in a clear, and comprehensive fashion, the contemporary scientific evidence on fibromyalgia . It will be of great service to patients and their health care providers; it should become "must reading" for interested third parties, such as insurers, who often need much help in understanding what fibromyalgia is.

Dr. Manfred Harth (Rheumatologist and Professor Emeritus, University of Western Ontario, London)

"If you have been belittled and ridiculed by family, friends, physicians, employers or attorneys who do not believe your fibromyalgia symptoms are real, this book is for you. Kevin P. White, M.D., Ph.D. restores the credibility and image of fibromyalgia by using scientific logic and examples of other well-known medical conditions to prove that you have a serious, life-impacting disease. White draws on his experience as a researcher in the field and treating physician to give you the ammunition you need to defend yourself against hurtful comments. Everything he states is backed by research. He offers tactful ways to get others to understand your symptoms and respect your physical limitations."

Kristin Thorson (President, American Fibromyalgia Syndrome Association (AFSA); Editor, Fibromyalgia Network Journal)

"I LOVED THE BOOK. It is long overdue. Dr. White's dedication and concern for the FM community show in EACH and EVERY word he writes."

Jackie Yencha, Vice President
National Fibromyalgia Partnership (NFP)

"If you have ever been told by a doctor, friend, or family member that FM does not exist and that your symptoms are not real, then this is the book for you. It is one of the best books I have ever read on fibromyalgia, written by one of the most qualified doctors in the field.

The book is expertly written with superb examples and analogies to explain complex scientific points, making the text user friendly and fully accessible to anyone with no medical knowledge. He tackles all the arguments that critics throw at fibromyalgia and all his statements are well supported by scientific research. It brings together the wealth of knowledge we now have about FM and moulds it into a strong argument to legitimise what FM patients around the world have been saying for years. Fibromyalgia is real!

With this book on your shelf you will have the ammunition to defend yourself against any onslaught from any person who says FM does not exist. It will certainly be taking up a space on my bookshelf."

Kathy Longley (Chief Editor, Fibromyalgia
Association of the United Kingdom)

"This insightful book is a valuable tool for lawyers who are prosecuting personal injury actions and long-term disability claims based on a condition that remains poorly understood by both the bench and bar. The detailed index and glossary make it a useful resource to bring right into the courtroom."

Ann Marie Frauts (personal injury lawyer; senior
partner, Frauts & Dobbie Attorneys at Law)

"Great strides have been made in the science of fibromyalgia during the past two decades, yet a great many people, both lay and medical, still fail to understand the breadth and significance of discoveries made. With his own impressive track record in FM research, Kevin White, M.D., Ph.D., is uniquely qualified to make an articulate and authoritative case for the legitimacy of FM. White's new book, *Breaking Thru the Fibro Fog*, is a must-read for anyone with a serious interest in fibromyalgia."

Tamara K. Liller
President & Director of Publications
National Fibromyalgia Partnership, Inc.
[a 501(3)(c) non-profit organization]

"A very well-written user-friendly book that effectively refutes the anti-fibromyalgia critics and gives much needed legitimacy to these long-suffering patients."

Fred Friedberg, PhD
President, International Association for Chronic Fatigue Syndrome

"Who should, or will read this book? Clearly, patients with fibromyalgia will wish to read it; but others on that list might include those who argue against the validity of this condition, family members who now perceive unexpected cracks in their shields, employers faced with an illness which they fear could affect the bottom line, politicians who are recognizing an illness that affects a large proportion of their constituents, lawyers on either side of controversial issues, and judges required to weigh the arguments in order to make decisions which fairly meet the dictates of law.

It is yet to be seen how history will view this book, but the first step in that process is for history to read its pages and digest its thoughts."

I. Jon Russell, MD, PhD
University of Texas Health Science Center at San Antonio Faculty
Retired Master, American College of Rheumatology
Editor, Journal of Musculoskeletal Pain
Coauthor, Fibromyalgia Helpbook

DEDICATIONS

This book is dedicated to the millions around the world who have fibromyalgia and have had to suffer in silence. May you now be heard!

And it is especially dedicated to my sister, Barbara. Thanks for everything you do.

ACKNOWLEDGMENTS

I have many to thank.

A sincere *thank you* goes to the countless people who helped me by reading this book prior to its publication to provide valuable feedback. Thank you especially to Dr. Manfred Harth, who has been a mentor to me throughout my professional career, and whose undying support of fibromyalgia patients helped me to develop mine; and to Dr. Jon Russell, another tireless FM advocate and researcher, whose assistance has been pivotal to this book being published.

Thank you to Darlene Steele, whose successful fight against fibro can serve as an inspiration to all, and whose help with this book really helped to bring it to final fruition. Thanks to Kristin Thorson and the American Fibromyalgia Syndrome Association, who have supported me in so many ways throughout the latter stages of this book's preparation, and to Tammy Liller and the National Fibromyalgia Partnership. Thanks also to Jim Asher, Joseé Lemay, and (at Ink Tree Marketing) Denise Hamilton for your continuous guidance in the publication of this book, and to Steve Matthews and Gord Nudds for your assistance with printing and distribution. And thanks to my wife and children for putting up with me throughout the countless hours I spent at my computer over the past 18 months as this book was written and revised.

ABOUT THE BOOK

Did you know that fibromyalgia is more common in Bangladesh and Pakistan than in any country in North America or Western Europe?

So much for the argument some critics use that fibromyalgia only exists because of wealthy western world insurance and compensation programs.

Fibromyalgia (FM) is a long-term, often disabling disease that affects up to one in ten women and one in sixty males over the course of their lifetimes; and yet many – including many in the healthcare and legal professions – fail to accept that it even exists, or that it can possibly be as disabling as patients say. Over the years, this has led to tremendous hardship for FM sufferers, as they struggle to make others, sometimes their own families and friends, sometimes their employer or own doctor, believe them.

This book is for all of you; and for those who love you; for those who employ you; for all the doctors and lawyers and others who seek to defend you and your rights; and for those who just want to read what the scientific evidence is and then decide for themselves. It contains not only clear, detailed explanations, but scientific references, a glossary of terms, a list of referenced authors, and an index to aid those who really want to explore the science behind this disease.

Fibromyalgia is real. This book should leave no room for doubt.

ABOUT THE AUTHOR

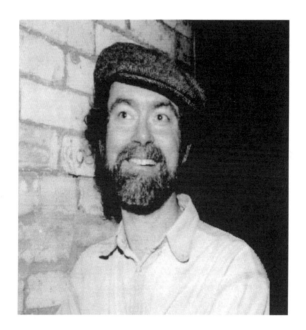

With a medical degree, training in two specialties and a further doctoral (Ph.D.) degree in medical research, Dr. White has been an internationally recognized expert in fibromyalgia treatment and research, fibromyalgia patient advocate, and former university Teacher of the Year. Now retired from active practice, he has turned to writing, having already written four novels, nine children's books, a book of inspirational essays and, as a singer-songwriter and multi-instrumentalist, over 400 songs. In this newest book, Dr. White returns to his roots in medical practice and research, trying to help millions of fibromyalgia sufferers with a book that, once and for all, tells all that FM really is real.

ABOUT THE BOOK'S COVER

The cover was designed by Darlene Steele, an amazing woman who epitomizes what this book is all about. She was an extremely busy office manager overseeing dozens of employees and operations while raising two daughters all on her own when, five years ago, she suddenly developed fibromyalgia and became unable to function in the workplace. Instead of giving up she, like Dr. White, turned to writing; and it was through a newspaper article announcing the release of one of her books that Dr. White learned her story. Finding out that she had designed the covers of her own book entirely herself, Dr. White asked her to design the cover to this book; and seeing the result, all his books. Though Ms. Steele still cannot function in a demanding workforce, it is clear that her brilliance and creativity are far too special to be wasted.

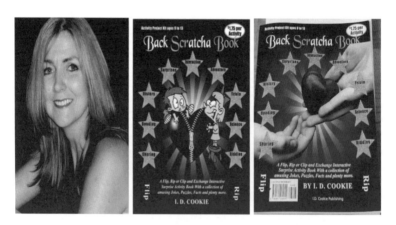

Darlene Steele (pen name I. D. Cookie) and one of her own books.
Darlene's books (under the pen name I. D. Cookie) are available at
www.wortleyroadbooks.com and www.backscratchabook.com

FOREWORD
by I. Jon Russell, M.D., Ph.D.

How interesting it would have been to listen in on the conversations of Greek or Roman philosophers as they offered to their students contemporary knowledge gleaned from careful observation and study. Our culture pretends to be so advanced over those that came before us, but the likelihood is that the concerns of those ancient peoples were not very different from our own.

In this book, the reader can almost voyeuristically listen as Kevin White, M.D., Ph.D. explains fibromyalgia to his patients. As he addresses each symptom or finding, the good doctor uses illustrations that he knows will be familiar. The listener is struck by the hominess of the physician's domestic experience. On one occasion he is folding laundry, while on another, the focus is on the severity of his own pain sustained in an accidental injury.

It should come as no surprise that Dr. White speaks with more than one voice in different parts of the book. In fact, he has at least three voices and he uses two of them in these pages, depending on what is needed. In one chapter, the reader experiences the down-to-earth clinician voice (M.D.) trying to help his patient understand chronic widespread pain or dysfunctional, non-restorative sleep. In another, the reader will encounter the authoritative scientific voice (Ph.D.) describing the meaning of sophisticated research findings. Dr. White's scientific training and experience comes through when he is quoting original sources and teaching through the presentation of research findings. Dr. White knows this material so well because he conducted much of the research himself. It was he who studied the epidemiology of fibromyalgia in Canada. It was he who quieted the critics when they claimed that it is medically harmful to make the diagnosis of fibromyalgia. It was he who discovered the high prevalence of fibromyalgia in the Amish people of Canada.

Dr. White's third voice, by the way, is that of a folk singer who has put to music many interesting vignettes from Canadian history. Look it up on any internet search engine and listen to one of his CD albums. Bet you can't stop with just one.

There are now many books on the market that present the scope of fibromyalgia in the world today. Each offers something unique to the reader. So, why is this book needed and why will it find an important place in the field? To this question, there are many answers. Only a few medical topics have suffered so much from bias and misunderstanding as fibromyalgia, but attitudes are changing. Perhaps for that reason, few fields in medicine are advancing at the rapid rate we now observe with fibromyalgia. Every new research finding must be examined carefully for relevance and importance. All of the new data require expert integration and then explanation.

Who should, or will read this book? Clearly, patients with fibromyalgia will wish to read it but others on that list might include those who argue against the validity of this condition, family members who now perceive unexpected cracks in their shields, employers faced with an illness which they fear could affect the bottom line, politicians who are recognizing an illness that affects a large proportion of their constituents, lawyers on either side of controversial issues, and judges required to weigh the arguments in order to make decisions which fairly meet the dictates of law.

It is yet to be seen how history will view this book but, the first step in that process is for history to read its pages and digest its thoughts.

I. Jon Russell, M.D., Ph.D.
University of Texas Health Science Center at San Antonio Faculty
Retired Master, American College of Rheumatology
Editor, Journal of Musculoskeletal Pain
Coauthor, Fibromyalgia Helpbook

CONTENTS

PART I
FIBROMYALGIA: WHAT IT IS & ISN'T

PART II
TWELVE SCIENTIFIC REASONS FIBROMYALGIA IS REAL

PART III
TRAUMA, DISABILITY AND DYLAN

SUPPLEMENTARY MATERIALS

INTRODUCTION, BY DR. WHITE
WHY I'M WRITING THIS

I was seven years into my medical training towards becoming a practicing pain specialist before I ever heard the term *fibrositis*. Not once did I recall it having been mentioned in medical school or during my residency training in Internal Medicine, until I went to a 3-day symposium in Napa, California, on arthritis and rheumatism. The lecture on fibrositis was the last one given, over the final lunch. Many attending the symposium had already left. I suspect that those who hadn't left mostly had stayed for the fancy lunch, rather than for the lecture. I listened to what this specialist was saying and, I am sorry to say, at some level thought he was some sort of snake oil salesman, trying to sell me on some disease without any physical or laboratory signs, and without any changes apparent on X-ray, CAT scan, MRI or any other imaging technique. It sounded a bit like hocus-pocus to me.

It was almost a year later, months into my own specialty training in Rheumatology (specializing in diseases of the musculoskeletal system, like bones and joints) that I saw my first 'fibrositis' patient, though now the disorder was more often called 'fibromyalgia'. Over the next ten years of training and my own practice, I probably saw two to three thousand more such patients; and though different in some ways, there were so many things they all had in common... the pain everywhere; the extreme fatigue; the poor sleep; the problems with memory.

Over this time, I had obtained a second doctoral degree (Ph.D.) in medical research, to go along with my M.D. degree, so I had developed into a pretty critical thinker. That critical thinking led me to really look into this condition that I wasn't sure I believed in or not. Over time, I came to believe in it more and more. And, over time, I came to see how fibromyalgia patients were being denied so many rights afforded patients with other painful conditions, like arthritis and heart disease. Many were denied disability payments when they became unable to work. Many essentially were told by doctors and

14

insurance companies and lawyers and judges and friends and family members that they just needed to "snap out of it." Repeatedly, I read opinion papers – almost exclusively written by doctors who hadn't done research in the area or, sometimes, in ANY area - that fibromyalgia wasn't real; that doctors who supported this diagnosis were doing more harm than good. Finally, I wrote an opinion paper myself, called **Fibromyalgia: The Answer Is Blowin' in the Wind** (Journal of Rheumatology, 2004;31: 636-9), in which I poked holes in every single one of the arguments that I had heard raised against fibromyalgia. Of all the scientific papers and book chapters and other medical writings I have done to date, I consider that one opinion paper the crowning accomplishment of my career. I see it everywhere on the internet. In fact, if you Google search my name, that paper is probably the very first thing that will appear.

This book is that opinion paper expanded, and written in a way such that patients and doctors and lawyers and loved ones of patients and anyone else who wants to find out why fibromyalgia (FM) truly exists can really delve into it. I have included the scientific references on which I base my arguments and conclusions, including many scientific papers I published myself.

Writing this book has been difficult, because of the diverse audience this book is intended for. I have wanted, on one hand, to make it easy to read, even for those with no or next to no medical or scientific background. On the other hand, I also want it to be informative and of use to doctors, lawyers, and other professionals who want to delve more into the science of what I'm writing (hence, the glossary of terms, index, lists of referenced researchers and authors, and a complete list of references to papers and study results that have been published in various scientific journals). I hope that I have achieved that delicate balance, so everyone can read and get something useful from this. My ultimate goal for this book is that it will help those with fibromyalgia get back some of the respect and rights that every single person deserves.

Kevin P. White, M.D., Ph.D.

PART 1

FIBROMYALGIA:

WHAT IT IS

AND

WHAT IT ISN'T

CHAPTER 1

WHAT IS FIBROSITIS/FIBROMYALGIA?

Fibrositis and *fibromyalgia* (FM) are the exact same thing. *Fibrositis* is an older term that was coined in 1904 by Dr. William Gowers(1).[*] This term literally means 'inflammation in fibrous tissues'; fibrous tissues being, for example, *tendons* that connect muscles to bone, and *fascia*, which is a nerve-rich, thin, sac-like structure that surrounds every muscle, kind of like slippery Saran wrap.

Meanwhile, the term *fibromyalgia* means 'pain in muscles and fibrous tissues'. The defining characteristic of all fibromyalgia patients, therefore, is pain that, for years, was believed to originate in muscles, fibrous tissues, or both. What all this means it that, if you don't have pain, <u>by definition</u> you don't have fibromyalgia as it currently is defined.

But fibromyalgia (which I will abbreviate to FM) is not just pain in your left finger and right knee. People with fibromyalgia have widespread pain, pain that seems to affect their muscles everywhere, or almost everywhere. Roughly half of FM patients say that they hurt all over(2). To some who don't have FM, this sounds strange: how can someone possibly hurt all over? But to them I ask: have you ever had a really bad flu where you ached all over? Maybe you also had a splitting headache, and felt so wiped out and weak you could barely stand. In a nutshell, THAT is how most patients with FM feel... like they have the worst flu of their life; and, worst of all, it virtually NEVER goes away.

The pain of FM frequently is accompanied by other muscle problems as well, like severe muscle stiffness, especially in the morning, but also after the person does

---

[*] The number (1) here refers to a scientific paper or book, listed at the end of the book, in the section called References, where you can find evidence that the statement I have just made is true.

something that they used to do easily, like getting dressed(2), and sometimes lasting all day(3).

Additional sources of pain are headaches, eye pain, sore throat, and abdominal and pelvic pain. A minority of patients have considerable discomfort when they pass urine. Many have regular abdominal (belly) cramps. And so on.

The bottom line is this: persons with fibromyalgia hurt, seemingly everywhere or almost everywhere.

But, technically, FM is more than just widespread pain. First the pain must be chronic, which means 'long-lasting'; and, by this, I mean having lasted at least three months. This is to distinguish it from that really bad flu I mentioned earlier.

And, to meet the current medical definition of FM, besides widespread pain, someone also needs to be tender in characteristic areas when a doctor or some other diagnostician (like a therapist) pushes on these points relatively lightly with their thumb. How this is done will be covered in the next chapter.

But FM is even more than chronic widespread pain and tenderness. It also includes a host of other symptoms that may or may not be present in any given patient. This collection of symptoms has led some to call the condition *fibromyalgia syndrome*.

But what is a syndrome? The best analogy I can come up with is that FM is kind of like a city bus. Have you ever ridden the same bus every day at the same time over an extended period of time, for example, to go to school or to work? Maybe this was before you had a car; or after you no longer could afford to keep one.

Pretend, if you will, that you get on the same bus at the same place and same time every day. Next, for the sake of this analogy, let's pretend that the driver is always the same. Let's also say that there are a few passengers who are VIRTUALLY ALWAYS on the bus at the same time you are riding it: perhaps there's an old woman who always sits in the third row; a middle-aged man with a brief case; and a kid who sits in the back. In addition, there are a few people who USUALLY are on the bus; not every day, but most days; there are some who OFTEN are on the bus, maybe 30% of the time; and finally, there are some you recognize, but who are only on the bus OCCASIONALLY.

Fibromyalgia syndrome is kind of like that. The DRIVER of the fibro bus is chronic widespread pain. If a person doesn't have pain, they don't have fibromyalgia... they must be riding some other bus, because pain is the defining characteristic of fibromyalgia. The passengers who are VIRTUALLY ALWAYS on the bus are the characteristic tender points; occasionally, we see a person who has all the symptoms of FM but who isn't that tender, but this is quite uncommon. In addition, fatigue and poor sleep are almost always a problem. Other symptoms that USUALLY are present are problems with concentration and short-term memory – something that has been called the *fibro fog*(4). And so on. A more complete list of fibromyalgia symptoms is this:

MUST BE PRESENT (for it to truly be FM, as it is currently defined; this will be explained in greater detail in the next chapter)
- Chronic widespread pain
- Chronic widespread body tenderness

VIRTUALLY ALWAYS PRESENT
- Debilitating (disabling) fatigue
- Poor (non-restorative) sleep (you wake up feeling worse than when you went to bed)

ALMOST ALWAYS PRESENT
- Problems with short-term memory
- Problems with concentration
- Headaches

- Migraine headaches

OFTEN PRESENT

- Diarrhoea; constipation; or diarrhoea alternating with constipation (commonly called *irritable bowel*)
- Crampy abdominal pain
- Abdominal bloating
- Pelvic discomfort
- Urinary urgency (having to go immediately) associated with discomfort
- Numbness and tingling, especially in the hands and feet
- Cold-induced whitish discoloration of the hands and feet (something that is called *Raynaud's phenomenon*)

Other less common symptoms can occur too, but it is beyond the scope of this book to go into them all. Suffice it to say that the bus analogy and the list of symptoms given above should give you a pretty good idea of what fibromyalgia is.

Some of the characteristic features of FM - like the debilitating fatigue, the poor sleep, and the fibro fog - have been reasonably well explained by the research that already has been done on FM. The association between FM and certain other symptoms, like the diarrhoea and hand discoloration, seem less intuitive, though our recent understanding of FM as more of a neurological than a musculoskeletal disease makes such connections more understandable. A lot more about this will come in later chapters.

Other Signs of Fibromyalgia

In addition to the characteristic fibromyalgia tender points, there are numerous other things that doctors may find when they perform a physical examination. For example, FM patients characteristically state that their worst areas include their neck and shoulders, and their low back and hips. Understandably, then, patients with FM often are diffusely tender throughout these regions, and many show decreased range of motion of the neck, shoulders and low back.

In addition to diffuse (widespread) tenderness in these areas, patients also frequently have something called *myofascial* (= muscle + fascia) *trigger points*(2;5). *Trigger points* should not be mistaken for tender points, though this error commonly is made by physicians and other examiners. A *tender point* is a point on the body surface that, when pushed upon by an examiner's thumb, causes pain directly under the thumb. A *trigger point*, on the other hand, is a point on the body surface that, when pushed upon by an examiner's thumb, causes pain that radiates (spreads) away from the point that is being pushed; for example, pushing on the mid trapezius muscle of the shoulder (half way between the neck and the tip of the shoulder) may cause pain to shoot up the neck and down the adjacent arm. This process of *triggering* is what Kellgren and Lewis described in their experiments in the 1930s(6-9).

Two additional physical findings commonly present in FM patients are skin-fold tenderness (literally, pinching the skin lightly causes severe pain) and something called *reactive hyperaemia*(2). Reactive hyperaemia (*hyperaemia* means: too much blood) most commonly is observed on the patient's back. After the doctor pushes down with his or her thumb and then lets go, the patient's skin becomes very red and warm, and will remain so for minutes or even hours afterwards, as opposed to returning to normal color and temperature within seconds, which is what happens in people without FM.

The importance of reactive hyperaemia is that it cannot possibly be faked.
Unfortunately, it is not seen in a significant enough majority of individuals with FM and not absent in enough people without FM to be considered diagnostic. Nonetheless, it can be a dramatic finding which often is directly over the patient's areas of greatest reported pain.

A *dolorimeter* or *algometer* (both of which literally mean 'a pain measuring device') is a small tool that doctors and therapists sometimes use to quantify a patient's level of

23

tissue tenderness. It is a spring-loaded device with a rubber end attached to a numerical dial; in essence, it looks kind of like a stop-watch with a rubber stopper sticking out on a short rod (see picture below). The examiner pushes the rubber end into the patient's muscle at a perpendicular angle, asking that patient to say when the pushing starts to hurt. The examiner then ceases pushing and records the level of pressure that was being applied when the patient first said it hurt. In fibromyalgia, patient pain thresholds are usually very, very low. In other words, even very light touch with a dolorimeter causes the patient to have pain.

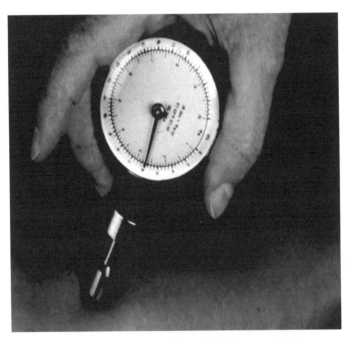

An algometer/dolorimeter measures a patient's degree of tenderness

Decreased pain threshold on dolorimetry testing has been proposed as a more 'objective' physical finding than tenderness to an examiner's thumb, but dolorimetry testing may be less sensitive(2). Hence, most FM experts recommend that doctors use their thumb instead of a dolorimeter when making the diagnosis of FM.

Dolorimetry readings are sensitive to numerous factors, like the size of the dolorimeter's rubber foot plate, the dolorimeter's scale length (for example, can pressure readings be measured just to 5 kg pressure or can they be measured as high as 7 kg or even 9 kg?) and the rate at which dolorimeter pressure is applied(10-12); for example, does the doctor push down slowly or really quickly? What all this means is that any doctor who insists that a patient's previously-made diagnosis of FM is wrong because no dolorimeter was used, themselves are wrong. At this time, the only validated role dolorimeters have, at least with respect to FM, is in scientific research.

Who Gets FM?

Women appear to be more likely to get FM than men, but both genders get it. In our own survey of almost 3300 adults living in London, Ontario, Canada, we confirmed the diagnosis in roughly one in twenty women and about one in sixty men(13). Most had never been diagnosed. In fact, though it hopefully has improved over time, the average duration of symptoms before someone with FM ever even gets to see an appropriate specialist who could diagnose it, has been as long as between 5 and 8 years(3;14-16).

People of all ages can get it, including children(17); but it is most commonly first diagnosed in those who are in their thirties through fifties(13).

Several patterns of disease onset have been described. One pattern is a slow, insidious onset without any precipitating event. A second pattern of onset is much more sudden (acute), often appearing to have been precipitated by something like an injury. There are those who suggest that FM often is caused by some form of injury(18;19). And a small percentage of cases seem to start after some sort of fever-associated illness (presumably an infection), though whether any true relationship exists remains unproven(20;21).

FM may present in association with a variety of psychiatric illnesses. In several studies, FM patients have scored higher than controls (those without FM) on a variety of

25

psychometric scales[†] for anxiety, depression, and hypochondria(22-25). Some have interpreted this as evidence either that psychiatric illness causes FM, or that FM is a psychiatric illness(26;27). Extreme caution must be exercised when interpreting the results of these studies, however. First of all, patients with long-standing (chronic) pain, irrespective of the cause, will score abnormally high on a number of such psychometric tests when compared against those who are healthy(28), which may result in the tests being wrong, particularly when assessing for depression, hysteria and hypochondria(28;29). Second, the majority of patients with FM do not show significant differences in these psychometric scores relative to patients with some painful condition like rheumatoid arthritis(22;25). Third, the majority of FM patients seen in rheumatology clinics do not have a psychiatric illness(15;30). And fourth, there is evidence that psychiatric diagnoses in FM patients are related to health care-seeking behaviour, rather than to the illness itself(31). In other words, the ones with FM who are most likely to be sent to a specialist are those who are most psychologically distressed by it; which makes complete sense.

The evidence is as strong or stronger that FM is associated with a variety of other non-psychiatric disorders, with one study finding FM in 15% of 522 hospital in-patients on the Internal Medicine ward at a large Israeli hospital(32). FM frequently occurs in the setting of other rheumatic diseases. Somewhere between about 20% and 65% of rheumatology clinic patients with a very complex condition called primary *systemic lupus erythematosis* (SLE) meet the American College of Rheumatology (ACR) criteria for FM(33-35), and FM appears to be a common component of other arthritis conditions like rheumatoid arthritis(36), osteoarthritis(37), and psoriatic arthritis(38), among others. Men and women who are infected with the human immunodeficiency virus (HIV) that causes AIDS(39) or with human T cell lymphocytic virus type I(40), and women with excessively high hormone levels of either prolactin(41) or thyroid hormone(42) appear to have a significantly increased risk of FM. Women with high prolactin levels have a risk that is fifteen times as great as women without(41). Men with a condition called

---

[†] A psychometric scale is usually a questionnaire that asks the patient various questions about their mood, level of anxiety, and so on.

sleep apnea (where people actually stop breathing for very short periods, like several seconds, during sleep) might have an increased risk of FM, though the research is not entirely clear on this (43;44). And, though generally only seen in less than half of FM patients, several studies conducted worldwide over the past 15 years have documented an association between FM and joint hyper-mobility(45-49).

So, if FM commonly is present in people with other diseases, how about the reverse? How common are other conditions in people with FM? Despite the apparent associations between FM and various other illnesses in clinic studies, there have been no studies estimating the frequency of such illness in individuals with FM in the general community. However, since FM appears to be considerably more common than most of these other conditions, it may be that co-morbid (coincident) illness only affects a small percentage of the total FM population. If this seems contradictory to you, think of this analogy:

Patients with a condition like lupus commonly have FM just like grapes commonly have seeds. Yes, there are seedless grapes; but a large percentage of grapes have seeds. On the other hand, only a small percentage of all the seeds that exist in the world are inside a grape, just like only a small percentage of all those with FM have lupus.

The Course of Fibromyalgia

By definition, fibromyalgia is chronic, since the pain must have lasted at least 3 months for the condition to be diagnosed. But what happens long term? Suffice it to say that, if FM went away relatively quickly – for example, within a year or two – there would probably be no need for a book such as this; patients themselves would be less frustrated; and everyone else – from uncertain family members to employers and insurers – would be more supportive. Unfortunately, however, FM is much more chronic than this, with most patients having continued pain, fatigue, and other symptoms for years, if not indefinitely. The outlook seems somewhat less bleak in children and teenagers; but, with the exception of an Australian study in which 24% of patients had entered into clinical remission within 2 years of their initial assessment(50), at least in adults, complete remission is uncommon(51-57), and the response to treatment often is modest. That is not to say that all patients do poorly. But, as noted in Chapter 17, many become unable to continue working, and most experience major reductions in their activity level. It is the issue of disability that probably sparks the greatest degree of controversy over this condition, even among those who support the FM concept(51;52;58-62). The issue of trauma as a precipitator of FM takes on additional importance given the persistence of symptoms, so it has become a second major source of controversy. And, in response to these two issues, naysayers have flourished, as Chapter 3 will illustrate. One final issue that I will cover briefly here is the controversy over whether FM and chronic fatigue syndrome are the same condition, within the same spectrum of disorders, or quite distinct.

The FM versus CFS/ME Debate

It is not at all uncommon among support or advocacy groups to include both FM and *chronic fatigue syndrome* (CSF; also called *myalgic encephalomyelitis* or ME) in the group name. In Canada, for example, the CFS-FM Action Network provides advocacy, information and patient support to those with either CFS or FM. Similarly, in Australia, the various regional branches of the ME/CFS Society Inc. all provide information and support to those with FM too. This likely is because, in terms of how patients feel, the two conditions seem to have more similarities than differences.

As with FM, there is no single diagnostic test that is useful for diagnosing CSF. The first working definition of CFS that the Centre for Disease Control (CDC) in Atlanta, Georgia endorsed was published in 1988. This definition required that a patient fulfill one major and a number of minor criteria, most of which are very subjective symptoms (for example, joint pain) or non-specific physical signs (for example, fever)(63). Later sets of criteria, published in 1994 and 2005, similarly rely on patient symptoms rather than any hard physical findings(64;65). Although the case definition for CFS also requires that other potential causes of fatigue be excluded, it is very difficult to exclude FM because of the striking similarities between these two syndromes. Profound fatigue often is a major complaint among fibromyalgia patients. Diffuse muscle and joint pain is a frequent symptom of CFS, each being one of the 11 minor symptom criteria in the case definition. In fact, virtually every one of the minor symptom criteria for CFS is a frequent complaint among FM patients. And, although many consider CFS to be transmitted by an infectious agent, like a virus or bacterium, a flu-like or other infectious onset is not required by the 1988 CDC criteria. Moreover, as stated earlier, some cases of FM may begin after a febrile (fever-associated) illness.

Other similarities between FM and CFS are that each has no definitively known cause; there is no highly effective therapy for either syndrome; the symptoms in both tend to be chronic(long-term); and both conditions seem to be more common in women, including young women(66).

What is apparent is that current criteria do not differentiate these two disorders well(67;68). In other words, patients who meet one set of criteria often meet the other. Wysenbeek and his research associates evaluated 33 FM patients and found that 21% met the CDC criteria for CFS, as well(69). Hudson and his research partners similarly studied 33 rheumatology clinic patients with FM, and found that 14 (42%) met the full CDC criteria for CFS, and an additional 9 (27.3%) were within one minor symptom of meeting the CDC criteria(70). Goldenberg has identified similar high rates of concurrence between FM and CFS(71;72). And in our own study of 100 community cases of FM, roughly 60% of the females and 80% of the males with FM also met the case definition for CFS(68). What we also found is that those who met both sets of criteria reported a worse course, worse overall health, more dissatisfaction with health, more non-CFS symptoms, and greater disease impact than those who met the FM criteria alone. In other words, meeting both sets of criteria (for FM and CFS) means that you tend to feel worse and do more poorly; it doesn't really mean you have two separate diseases.

Of those who strictly meet the FM but not the CFS definition, and *vice versa*, there may be some underlying differences at a causative level. For example, Evengard and colleagues, and Russell and colleagues both found that FM patients, but not those with CFS, had elevated levels of a pain neurotransmitter called substance P in their spinal fluid(73;74). And, though not all research groups have found this, there MAY be an association between the retrovirus XMRV and CFS, an association not yet identified for FM(75). However, especially given the high degree of clinical similarity between the two conditions and how frequently a given person will meet both sets of criteria, it may be some time before the FM-CFS issue is resolved.

So... what is FM again?

FM is a condition in which patients have widespread, long-lasting pain (often everywhere), severe fatigue, sleep problems, and diffuse body tenderness, with other symptoms possible as well. It is fairly common, especially in women, but affects men and children too. It sometimes exists on its own, and sometimes at the same time as other conditions; either way, it can be and often is quite disabling. The next chapter will clarify how it is, or at least how it should be, diagnosed.

CHAPTER 2
MAKING THE DIAGNOSIS

I already have given you a bit of an idea about how fibromyalgia (FM) is diagnosed. The most important additional point that I will make in this chapter is that FM is not a diagnosis of exclusion. In other words, it is not a diagnosis that should be entertained only after extensive examination and testing has ruled out everything else. It is not a garbage pail diagnosis intended for patients whose symptoms doctors just cannot explain (for example, let's just throw it here). Nor should FM be considered just the end of a spectrum of the usual aches and pains we all feel, a suggestion one critic in particular has made repeatedly(76;77); this is a comment that I will address further later in this chapter. FM is a specific diagnosis that is made after the doctor has taken a thorough history and completed a thorough physical examination, looking specifically for the following:

- Chronic (= long-standing), widespread pain
- Debilitating fatigue
- Non-restorative (poor) sleep
- Other symptoms commonly associated with FM
- Diffuse body tenderness.

As stated in the preceding chapter, there now are classification criteria that were created largely for research purposes, but which have been widely utilized to diagnose FM in clinical practice. To meet the criteria, a patient must have:

- Chronic, widespread pain.
  - o 'Chronic' meaning no fewer than three months of pain; this is to distinguish it primarily from that horrible flu someone might have with which they ache all over.

31

o 'Widespread' meaning...

1. Above and below the waist, and...

2. Right and left side of the body, and...

3. Involving the limbs and the trunk.

AND

o Tenderness at no fewer than 11 of 18 specific fibromyalgia tender points. The 18 points include 9 points on the right side of the body and the same 9 points on the left side of the body; in other words, 9 symmetrical or mirror-image points.

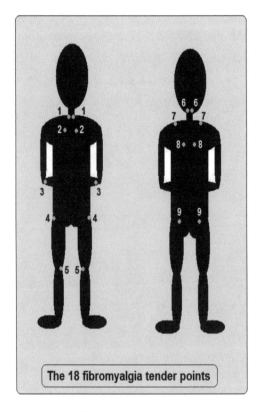

The 18 fibromyalgia tender points

o Specific locations of the fibromyalgia tender points are:

1. Near the base of the neck in the front.

2. Along the second rib, just before it joins the sternum (the breast bone).

3. Two centimetres past the elbow on the side of your 5th finger (your pinkie finger).

4. Just behind the bony part on the outer side of the hip (immediately behind the front pockets of your pants).

5. The inner fat pad of the knee.

6. The base of the skull as it meets the back of the neck, where the levator scapula muscle meets the skull.

7. The midpoint of the muscle (called the trapezius) that runs between the neck and the shoulder.

8. The upper, inner angle of the shoulder blade.

9. The upper, outer quadrant of the buttock.

Some have argued that the diagnosis of fibromyalgia should never be made, because there are no objective (visible and measurable) findings, either on physical examination or on laboratory testing, like obvious joint swelling or a marked elevation of some chemical in the blood. However, as I will discuss in several of the chapters in Part 2 of this book, this argument is extremely weak. A brief glimpse of one among many strong counter-arguments is this...

- Have you ever had a headache?
- Prove it.

The fact is: none of us can prove that we have headaches. And yet almost every one of us will have had one, at least once in our lifetime. Many people have headaches on a regular basis. But there is no objective evidence at all that headaches exist. Our technology just has not caught up with reality... we cannot detect headaches, at least not using any routine physical examination or clinical laboratory technique. If we held headaches up to the same level of zealous scrutiny to which some hold FM, we could never diagnose a headache. But does this make sense? Of course not.

But there will be much more on this later.

FM Is Not Diagnosed by Exclusion

I stated at the outset that FM is not a disorder that should be made only when all other possibilities are excluded. There are two major reasons for this. The first reason is:

- FM is a collection of symptoms that is different from that seen in other disorders.

There truly are very few conditions in which a patient says he or she hurts or aches all over, other than that terrible but short-lived flu I mentioned two pages ago. Occasionally, patients with leukaemia will report this; however, it is very rare that leukaemia will be missed diagnostically for very long.

Patients with arthritic conditions like rheumatoid arthritis (RA), osteoarthritis (OA) or lupus (SLE) rarely report aching all over. They may report hurting or having stiffness in multiple joints, such as several fingers, both wrists and both knees. However, it is uncommon that they say they ache all over. The exception to this is when individuals with one or more of these other conditions also have FM. And many patients with these other conditions do, in fact, also have FM. And this is the second reason that FM is not diagnosed when every other possible diagnosis has been eliminated. In short:

- FM can co-exist with other conditions.

As stated in the previous chapter, a significant minority (up to a third) of patients with rheumatoid arthritis (RA) will also meet the diagnostic/classification criteria for FM(36). They generally report more overall symptoms, worse pain, and worse fatigue than their RA counterparts who do not also have FM. Similarly, a sizeable minority of lupus (SLE) patients meet the ACR criteria for FM(33-35). And, as noted in the previous chapter, the list goes on. Having said this, most FM patients do not have RA, lupus or some other disease. This is because most of these other conditions are much less common than FM. For example, FM is approximately 10 times more common than RA, and approximately 100 times more common than lupus(52).

The essential point is that, irrespective of whatever other health conditions a person has, FM is diagnosed based upon whether or not that individual reports chronic, widespread, musculoskeletal pain and has widespread body tenderness. Further work-up to determine whether or not they have some other concomitant disorder or disorders sometimes is appropriate; but the findings of this work-up, whether positive or negative, do not alter the FM diagnosis itself. There may be instances in which the other condition is considered more important, in terms of which disorder to evaluate further and/or treat. But if you have RA and FM, or SLE and FM, or multiple sclerosis and FM, both conditions should be acknowledged.

Some might argue that the fact that FM commonly co-exists with other conditions is proof that it is not a distinct entity unto itself. But two strong counter-arguments to this are:

1. It often does exist on its own; and
2. Many other, well-accepted conditions commonly co-exist with others. Migraine headaches and pulmonary hypertension (elevated blood pressure in the blood vessels feeding the lungs) are two such examples; though both can exist alone, both also are common components of other diseases.

So again, FM is not a diagnosis that is made when you cannot find any other explanation for symptoms. It is diagnosed using scientifically-established criteria, following a comprehensive health interview and physical examination.

What About Control Points?

Some doctors like to use something called *control points* to show that someone doesn't have FM and is just faking. The use of such control points for this purpose is not at all appropriate(78-82), however, as I will explain in much greater detail in Chapter 11.

What About No Points?

Within the last few months, the American College of Rheumatology (ACR) has endorsed preliminary diagnostic criteria for FM that do not rely on a tender point examination(83). In fact, no examination of the patient is required at all. Instead, patients are asked questions about pain and where it is; about fatigue and whether or not they wake up refreshed; about cognitive symptoms like memory and concentration; and then about a whole host of other symptoms and how severe they are. Based upon a given patient's responses, they then are assigned a widespread pain index (WPI) score and a symptom severity (SS) score, and these scores are used to determine whether or not they have FM.

Of course, as with the original 1990 ACR criteria, they must have had symptoms for at least three months, and they cannot have any other disorder that might explain their symptoms. The authors acknowledge limitations of the study they utilized to generate these new criteria, and of the criteria themselves. They even, though clearly discrediting the use of tender points by excluding them in the new criteria, recommend that a tender point examination still be done.

The rationale behind these new criteria escapes me, largely for this reason: though many have argued over how accurate and useful the tender point exam is, as I will discuss again in Chapter 11, tenderness is a physical sign that is used for hundreds of other diseases and injuries; why is it suddenly suspect in FM? Numerous other strong arguments supporting the use of tender points have been made by Harth and Nielson(84).

A second issue is this: what advantage do these criteria present over the previous 1990 version? Obviously, there cannot be that much of an advantage if the authors themselves encourage examiners to still check for tender points.

A third point is that these criteria invariably lump together (1) persons with, for example, localized sciatica (pain from their low back into their buttock and thigh) that, in turn, causes them to have severe insomnia that, in turn, makes them wake up non-refreshed and feel profoundly fatigued, with (2) those who hurt and are tender to light touch all over. As an example of a condition where such lumping of extremes does not work, let's look at scleroderma. Scleroderma is a condition where patients have severe thickening of the skin (so thick it feels like wax). When this skin thickening is localized (for example, on the face or a single arm), it can be disfiguring. But when it is all over, it is associated with a whole host of other problems, like heart, lung, and kidney failure, that can be rapidly fatal. Specialists and researchers have made a point NOT to lump these two extremes of scleroderma together. So why do it now with FM?

Finally, for what other physical illness that is not diagnosed through some gold standard confirmatory lab test or imaging study have physical findings been removed from previously-established diagnostic criteria? None come to mind. My concern is that, by removing the physical exam from the evaluation of FM patients, these criteria run the risk of convincing even more physicians that FM is all in a patient's head. Although I hate even to think this, it is possible that the absence of any need to physically examine the patient to confirm FM even may be used by some specialists as an argument against them needing to see FM patients at all.

So... do I like the newly-proposed criteria?

In a word: No!

CHAPTER 3

FOURTEEN FALSEHOODS ABOUT FIBROMYALGIA (THAT NAYSAYERS ESPOUSE)

Fibromyalgia (FM) has been called "an illusionary entity(85)" and "a common non-entity(27)".   One author claims that FM is the result of "a long tradition of poor science(26)" and cites the opinion of another who had written: "In no other field have pseudoscientists flourished as prominently as in the field of medicine(86)". Fibromyalgia critics invariably use one of a number of arguments against its existence, all of which can be easily countered. In this chapter, I will list these so-called arguments against FM, and then go back over each one of them in a bit more detail, while providing brief counter-arguments. The chapters that follow this one will expand on the counter-arguments, providing references to indicate the research that has been published supporting the counter-arguments. It is important to note that **there is almost no scientific evidence supporting any of these arguments against FM.** Nonetheless, here they are:

1. Fibromyalgia is just the usual aches and pains everyone has, expressed in people who can't deal with them.

2. Fibromyalgia is a syndrome, not a disease.

3. Fibromyalgia only exists because of today's politically-correct bleeding-heart society.

4. Fibromyalgia only exists because of an overly-generous compensation system.

5. Fibromyalgia only exists because some people are lazy and want society to take care of them.

6. Fibromyalgia only exists because some doctors and researchers profit from its so-called 'existence'.

7. The way fibromyalgia is diagnosed is inherently flawed.

8. The way fibromyalgia initially was defined is inherently flawed.

9. All the symptoms of fibromyalgia are subjective.

10. Fibromyalgia is 100% subjective; there are no objective physical findings to suggest the disease is real.

11. There is no anatomical or physiological basis for fibromyalgia.

12. None of the objective physical or physiological findings in fibromyalgia are specific to this disorder.

13. No one has fibromyalgia until they are told they have it; if you removed the fibromyalgia label, these people wouldn't be nearly as 'sick'.

14. Fibromyalgia is a psychological, and not a physical disease.

Now let's go back over these fourteen anti-FM arguments in greater detail.

1. Fibromyalgia is just the usual aches and pains everyone has, expressed in people who can't deal with them.

In essence, this argument is that everyone has aches and pains, but most people live with these and just go on with their daily lives(76); a small percentage, however, just can't tolerate them. Maybe they have a low pain threshold. Maybe they are psychologically incapable of dealing with them. Maybe they see the opportunity for an easier life, not having to work while receiving compensation for so-called 'disability'. In the following chapters, I will refute these statements repeatedly. But several counter arguments for this one spring to mind immediately. First of all, you could say the same of conditions like migraine headaches and cluster headaches... I mean, almost everyone has headaches, don't they? What makes migraine headaches and cluster headaches so 'special' that they warrant a special designation, if FM doesn't? If we use the same logic some have used for FM, since everyone has headaches, aren't migraines and clusters just at the severe end of the usual headaches everyone has?

And what about polymyalgia rheumatica (PMR), a highly-accepted condition in which stiffness is prominent and little else... everyone gets a little stiff from time to time, don't they? Why do we treat stiffness in PMR?

Second, as I will demonstrate later in Chapter 15, several studies have shown that people with FM have no more psychological distress than others with similar levels of reported pain.

Third, studies have shown that people who just have aches and pains but not FM are, in fact, different in a number of both subjective and objective ways (in particular, see Chapters 7 and Chapters 9 through 12).

And fourth, any health care provider who has ever tried to get disability compensation approved for an FM patient will find that it is one of the most arduous, prolonged and demeaning processes any patient will ever have to go through; and the outcome is never certain... many are never compensated and end up living in abject poverty, losing their homes and families and friends and more. It is not, as some have claimed, an easy road at all. Chapter 17 details the many issues and obstacles related to disability in FM.

2. Fibromyalgia is a <u>syndrome</u> and not a <u>disease</u>.

With this argument, critics seem to be trying to make the point that syndromes are just a collection of symptoms, whereas diseases have real pathology. My first argument against this feeble attempt is this: look up the word *syndrome* in any dictionary or on the internet. The Oxford desk dictionary defines syndrome as *a group of characteristic symptoms of a disease*(87). Wikipedia, which tends to be quite exhaustive in its definitions, writes this:

In medicine and psychology, a **syndrome** is the association of several clinically recognizable features, signs (observed by a physician), symptoms (reported by the patient), phenomena or characteristics that often occur together, so that the presence of one feature alerts the physician to the presence of the others. In recent decades, the term has been used outside medicine to refer to a combination of phenomena seen in association.

The term *syndrome* derives from its Greek roots (σύνδρομος) and means literally "run together", as the features do. It is most often used to refer to the set of detectable characteristics when the reason that they occur together (the pathophysiology of the syndrome) has not yet been discovered(88).

And the 31st (2007) edition of Dorland's Illustrated Medical Dictionary(89) defines syndrome as "a combination of symptoms that either result from a single cause or occur together so commonly that they constitute a distinct clinical picture. See also disease and sickness".

Note that not one of these three sources, not even the two paragraphs supplied by Wikipedia, implies any lack of pathology; and that the first and last definitions actually use the word *disease* within the definition.

A second strong counter-argument to "FM is a syndrome not a disease" is this: look up the word *syndrome* in the index of any standard medical dictionary(89) or general medical textbook. What you will find is a long list of conditions in which the pathology is obvious, but for which the name still includes the word *syndrome*. Among the most common examples are Down's syndrome, Turner's syndrome, and the Syndrome of Inappropriate Antidiuretic Hormone (SIADH), all three of them conditions in which there is blatantly obvious and objective pathology (disease). Again, as I stated in Chapter 1, a syndrome is merely a collection of symptoms and signs that tend to run together like travellers on a city bus: these symptoms and signs can be as obvious and objective as a major deformity or death in infancy, or as 'subtle' as a mild headache; the term syndrome is open to both extremes and everything in between.

And the third counter-argument is for critics to read chapters 9 through 12 in this book, where any claim that there is no pathology in FM will be repeatedly and soundly thwarted.

3. Fibromyalgia only exists because of today's politically-correct, bleeding-heart society.

This is an extension of what I wrote about with the first anti-FM argument. Critics who utilize this line of ill-reasoning essentially believe that FM wouldn't exist if society just didn't tolerate it. But, as I note right away in the very next chapter, FM may have existed in biblical times; and certainly has existed since the mid 1900s, if not the mid 1800s, long before bleeding-heart societies with generous compensation systems were in existence (to see how 'generous' society used to be in the 1800s, just read Charles Dickens' famous novels *Oliver Twist* or *The Christmas Carol*). In addition, population studies have found FM to be more common in some very poor countries than wealthier ones, and in one particular population, the Amish, that specifically refuses to participate in ANY compensation system for religious reasons. Read Chapters 4 through 6 to explore all of this further.

4. Fibromyalgia only exists because of an overly-generous compensation system.

5. Fibromyalgia only exists because some people are lazy and want society to take care of them.

These two arguments are very similar, and many of the counter-arguments to the previous two statements apply here. Why, for example, would FM be more common in Bangladesh, arguably the poorest country in the World, than in prosperous and very society-conscious Sweden, if the generous compensation argument applies? And why would FM exist at all in the Amish? As with issue #3 above, the various counter-arguments are especially discussed in Chapters 4 through 6.

6. Fibromyalgia only exists because some doctors and researchers profit from its so-called 'existence'.

Believe it or not, I had this argument thrown at me by a doctor who was making hundreds of thousands of dollars every year doing *independent medical assessments* for insurance companies, when I often charged nothing for my dictated reports or for filling out forms.

Ask anyone you know in research if the following statement isn't true: scientific research in an area like FM pays little; in fact, most doctors who conduct such research would probably make much more if they devoted all their time to clinical versus research pursuits. Moreover, grounding one's research in a controversial area like fibromyalgia might even hurt one's career. Imagine a young FM researcher applying for a university faculty position at a medical school where the Chief of Medicine or the head of their division happens not to believe in FM.

7. The way fibromyalgia is diagnosed is inherently flawed.

8. The way fibromyalgia initially was defined is inherently flawed.

These arguments come back to the way doctors diagnose fibromyalgia using criteria, instead of a confirmatory blood test or X-ray or other scan. As stated in the first two chapters, FM is diagnosed when a patient has widespread pain and tenderness at specific areas. The way that these two criteria were decided upon was that researchers asked questions of, and examined over 260 patients already diagnosed as having FM by their specialist, and also asked questions of, and examined a similar number of patients with arthritis and other conditions believed NOT to have FM. The tautologic argument (as it is called, meaning a circular argument), is that this was a self-fulfilling prophecy. How did these doctors really know any of these patients really had FM? However, this method of establishing diagnostic or classification criteria is the same scientific method that has been used to develop classification criteria for every other disorder (including SLE and RA) for which they exist. If you find this confusing, rest assured that this argument and counter-argument will be clarified in Chapter 8.

9. All the symptoms of fibromyalgia are subjective.

This one is easiest of all to rebut, because all symptoms are, by definition, subjective. If you don't believe me, just do a Google search. Likely, the first entry you'll come to is the Wikipedia definition of symptom, which is as follows:

> A **symptom** (from Greek σύμπτωμα, "accident, misfortune, that which befalls", from συμπίπτω, "I befall", from συν- "together, with" + πίπτω, "I fall") is a departure from normal function or feeling which is noticed by a patient, indicating the presence of disease or abnormality. A symptom is subjective, observed by the patient, and not measured(90).

Or, if you would like a more scientific or academic reference, check out Dorland's Illustrated Medical Dictionary, 27th Edition, where a symptom is defined as "any subjective evidence of disease or of a patient's condition, i.e., such evidence as perceived by the patient; a change in a patient's condition indicative of some bodily or mental state."

I'm sorry, but any doctor who uses the "all the symptoms of fibromyalgia are subjective" argument needs to review their first-year medical school notes and/or buy and use a dictionary.

10. Fibromyalgia is 100% subjective; there are no objective physical findings to suggest the disease is real.

The argument here is that people with FM don't have a rash or measurable high fever or anything else that can be seen (actually visualized) and/or measured by the examining doctor. But there are many other highly-accepted conditions for which the same can be said (see Chapters 12 and 13). And, more important, in fact, is that there ARE observable and measurable physical findings in many FM patients. Most doctors don't know about them, so they don't look for them. They also are non-specific (meaning that people with other conditions also can have them); but they still are abnormal, indicating the presence of illness (see Chapter 11). And their lack of specificity for FM also is no argument, as this applies to most physical and laboratory findings in most diseases (see Chapter 12).

11. There is no anatomical or physiological basis for fibromyalgia.

In other words, if you do x-rays and routine blood tests on these patients, they all come back normal or unrelated to the patient's pain. Okay... this is true. However, if you do tests beyond the routine blood-work and imaging that most doctors know of, in fact, there are dozens and dozens of abnormalities that have been documented repeatedly in FM patients. And many of these abnormalities make perfect sense, given the symptoms FM patients report. Chapters 9 and 10 are all about this.

12. None of the objective physical or physiological findings in fibromyalgia are specific to this disorder.

Again, what critics are saying here is that none of the various things you do find wrong in a fibromyalgia patient are unique to fibromyalgia... so they are useless in justifying the condition. But, as I explain in detail in Chapter 12, this is true of almost everything. Virtually none of the physical findings your doctor looks for or routine blood tests your doctor orders are very specific for anything. You have a fever? So what... fevers aren't specific. Neither are 99% of rashes. Does this mean you ignore these signs? Of course not! This argument against fibromyalgia is pretty lame.

13. No one has fibromyalgia until they are told they have it; if you removed the fibromyalgia label, these people wouldn't be nearly as 'sick'.

One particular author seems to really like this one(76;91). He argues that people with FM wouldn't be nearly as sick if you just told them they weren't sick. First, I challenge him to try this, see the patients a second time maybe a year later, and then truthfully report on the results of his approach. And second, this already has been looked at in a large population study... and no, this was not the case at all(92). Read about all this in Chapter 14.

And, finally:

14. Fibromyalgia is a psychological, and not a physical, disease.

In other words, FM patients are just depressed, or anxious, or both... or they are just hypochondriacs. There are numerous counter-arguments against this one (see Chapter 15), including the fact that many patients with FM, when tested, show no evidence at all of depression, anxiety, hypochondria, or any other psychological illness. But the major point to be made here is that NO ILLNESS is 100% physical; and NO ILLNESS is 100% psychological. The physical illness vs. psychological illness dichotomy has been scientifically, thoroughly debunked!

Read on to have all these 14 counter-arguments expanded upon and scientifically justified in Part 2, Chapters 4 through 15. In Part 3, Chapter 16 specifically addresses the issue of post-traumatic fibromyalgia (FM that starts immediately following an accident of some kind), and Chapter 17 the issues of disability and disability assessments in FM. Chapter 18 wraps things up by going way back to the beginning, where it all started for me with a famous song by Bob Dylan.

PART 2

TWELVE
SCIENTIFIC REASONS

FIBROMYALGIA IS REAL

CHAPTER 4: REASON #1
FIBROMYALGIA IS <u>NOT</u> A NEW DISEASE

Among the various arguments that critics of the fibrositis/fibromyalgia concept use is that it only has come into existence because of current trends towards political correctness, in which society strives to include and accept virtually everyone, irrespective of what a person does or believes. Behaviours and beliefs that would not have been tolerated even 20 years ago are now politely smiled upon; or, at the very least, not criticized. There are support groups for everything. And society is instructed to be supportive, as well.

Hence, the argument goes, whereas 100 years ago, no one could get away with staying in bed all day, complaining of hurting everywhere and being too tired, because there were chores and other activities that just had to be done, today they have been afforded an acceptable 'out'. All someone needs to do is say that they have some disease that makes them so, and everyone will bend over backwards to accept them and it.

But listen to this: fibromyalgia <u>may</u> have existed since biblical times, with evidence supporting this claim identifiable in the Bible itself. In the Book of Job is written: *'and wearisome nights are anointed to me. When I lie down, I say, when shall I arise, and the night be gone? And I am full of tossings to and fro unto the dawning of the day... and the days of affliction have taken hold upon me. My bones are pierced in me in the night season; and my sinews take no rest. '*(93) Could this be describing FM? Now, I'll admit that this is weak supportive evidence; but it raises the possibility that FM has been with us since antiquity.

And there's more. Hans Christian Anderson also likely described fibromyalgia in his famous story 'The Princess and the Pea', when he wrote: *'In the morning they asked her how she had slept. "Dreadfully!" said the princess. "I hardly got a wink of sleep all night! Goodness knows what can have been in the bed! There was something hard in it, and now I m just black and blue all over! It's really dreadful! Only a real princess could be so tender as that."* (94) Here again is described poor sleep associated with widespread pain and/or tenderness.

There is considerable evidence that other, non-fictional individuals in history might have had FM. Alfred Nobel, who lived from 1833 to 1896, was a Swedish chemist, engineer, innovator, and the owner of a large weapons manufacturing company. Over his lifetime, he held 355 different patents, of which his most famous was dynamite. Upon his death, at the age of 63, it was his enormous fortune that instituted the Nobel Prizes, which are awarded annually even today, to world leaders in a variety of fields like science and literature, and include (somewhat ironically, I'd suggest, for the father of dynamite) the famous Nobel Peace Prize. Interestingly, despite having lived and died more than one hundred years ago, Nobel very well might have had FM. Why? Because, in numerous letters that he wrote over his lifetime to Sophie Hess, a woman he loved but never married, letters currently on display at the Nobel Institute in Stockholm, Alfred Nobel repeatedly mentions his recurrent headaches and chronic widespread pain. That he lived to the age of 63 without joint deformities argues against a diagnosis like rheumatoid arthritis; and that his pain was diffuse and chronic argues against diseases like osteoarthritis and gout. Of course, FM was never officially diagnosed while he was alive, because the condition hadn't even been recognized yet. But if a pain specialist of today heard someone describe the same diffuse pain, many if not most would consider FM high on their list of possibilities.

Similarly, Florence Nightingale, whom many would call the 'mother of modern nursing', herself was wracked by 'spinal pain', severe fatigue and insomnia for at least 40 years before her death in 1910, at the age of ninety. Presuming that spinal pain might have included pain elsewhere, she too may have had FM.

And you can go back even more than one thousand years ago to find possible FM. For if you visit Aachen, the westernmost city in Germany, you will find a monument to Charlemagne, one of the first Emperors of the Holy Roman Empire, who lived during the 8th and 9th century. There you will read how Charlemagne used to come to spend his winters in Aachen, because of its hot sulphur springs, which he did to relieve his chronic generalized pain. He did so until his death, at the then ripe old age of 72 years.

In fact, though the term *fibrositis* first was used by Dr. William Gowers in a paper he wrote on low back pain in 1904(1), to give a name to what he perceived was localized inflammation within muscles and fibrous tissues in the back, the concept of chronic (long-lasting) diffuse pain originating in muscles has been with us for centuries(84;95-97). Among the earliest scientific reports are some from the mid 1800s, especially in the German medical literature. In those early reports, pain was thought to be related to areas of muscle hardness(96;97) or muscle calluses(98) that doctors could feel, and that were very tender when pushed upon. The concept of inflammation within muscle and fibrous tissues initially was supported by a report by Stockman, in which he described inflammatory changes in "white fibrous tissue" of patients with "chronic rheumatism"(99). This finding was not reproduced in several subsequent studies, however, and the inflammatory focus hypothesis gradually was discarded(100;101); with it, went the name *fibrositis*, not to resurface until the mid 1970s in any meaningful way.

In the meantime, however, the concept that widespread pain could originate within small areas in deep tissue was supported by several studies that were conducted by the researchers Kellgren and Lewis, starting in the 1930s, with publications describing this spanning almost two decades(6-9;101;102). In their early studies, Kellgren and Lewis used blindfolded volunteers, on whom they demonstrated that injecting saline (salt water) into muscles and tendons could result in pain that radiated out from the injected site to distant parts of the body; not only that, but the distribution of the radiated pain caused by injecting a specific site was consistent from person to person. The pain also was associated with other characteristics like *referred tenderness* (meaning that these people were tender not only at the original site of injection, but also wherever else they had pain) and muscle spasms. So called *trigger points*(103), these characteristic sites of deep structure tenderness became part of a disorder ultimately called *myofascial pain syndrome* (MPS)[‡].

It was in the 1970s that two Canadian researchers, Moldofsky and Smythe, resuscitated the name *fibrositis* based upon several studies that revealed a correlation between abnormal sleep patterns and both chronic, widespread pain and characteristic points of body tenderness(104-107). In patients with chronic, widespread pain, and in healthy individuals undergoing experimentally-induced sleep deprivation involving the fourth of five stages of sleep, they identified what they called "an anomalous intrusion of alpha rhythms" into the normal brain wave (electroencephalographic, EEG) pattern of stage 4 delta wave activity. Moreover, 24 hours of experimental deprivation of stage 4 sleep (also called *stage IV sleep*), but not other stages, resulted in widespread pain and tenderness. They proposed that the label *fibrositis* be restricted to individuals with widespread pain and a non-restorative sleep pattern(108). Note that the scientific association between poor sleep and fibromyalgia will be discussed at great length in later chapters, especially Chapter 10.

In the late 1970s and 1980s, several research groups attempted to characterize the syndrome called *fibrositis* as it existed in rheumatology (arthritis) clinics, resulting in several additional sets of diagnostic criteria(3;14;15;108). Ultimately, the term *fibrositis* was changed to *fibromyalgia* (which means 'pain in muscles and fibrous tissues') to more accurately describe the condition, a name that persists to this day. The former term, after all, described an inflammatory process that no one ever had been able to confirm.

Finally, in 1990, the Fibromyalgia Multicentre Criteria Committee, under the auspices of the American College of Rheumatology (ACR), published criteria for FM that included a requirement for at least three months of widespread pain, and body tenderness at a

---

[‡] Please recall that the word 'myofascial' means originating in muscle and fascia (the lining around the muscle).

sufficient number of characteristic *tender points*(81). These criteria were selected, by consensus, based upon the results of a large, multi-centre study of approximately 265 patients previously diagnosed by their rheumatologist as having FM, and a similar number of patients, matched by age and sex, who previously had been determined not to have FM(81). These criteria, and the name *fibromyalgia* or *fibromyalgia syndrome*, persist to this day, both in clinical practice and for research purposes, even though many doctors make the diagnosis of FM without using them(109;110).

The name *fibromyalgia*, therefore, is relatively new. But the condition itself possibly has existed for thousands of years, and definitely for well over one hundred(84;95-97), long before the current climate of political correctness could have had any influential effect. So, to the critics who think that FM is merely a manifestation of all-inclusive, politically-correct modern times: history says otherwise!

CHAPTER 5: REASON 2
IT'S EVERYWHERE

Few, if any, would argue that fibromyalgia (FM) is uncommon. However, a frequently used critique among FM adversaries is that FM merely exists because there are disability insurance and compensation systems in place to support such individuals(111;112). The corollary to this is that FM would not exist if such individuals still were forced to work to survive.

However, there are several counter-arguments to this. One has just been reviewed in the previous chapter: chronic, widespread pain (and so, likely fibromyalgia) has been with us for at least a century, if not thousands of years, existing long before disability insurance and compensation systems came into being. Insurance systems cannot have 'created' FM if FM came first.

A second argument to counter the critics is that, although such systems now do exist, it is by no means easy for many FM patients to receive the disability payments they need to financially survive, thanks both to insurers restricting payments in the absence of clear evidence of disease or injury and disability (which is often hard to prove, and especially difficult in someone with no hard physical findings), and to the zealousness of critics who offer anti-FM arguments while ignoring the mountains of published evidence countering their oftentimes inflammatory opinions(26;27;76;85;91;98;111-114). One ill-informed judge in the Canadian province of Alberta characterized FM "as a court-driven ailment that has mushroomed into big business for plaintiffs"(115). And a leading FM researcher and proponent of the FM concept has argued that the diagnosis of FM should not be made in medicolegal settings (for example, when someone is bringing an insurance company to court in their fight for disability payments), both because of difficulties interpreting the tender point examination, and because of the escalating compensation claims and costs related to this disorder(60;62). From personal

57

experience assisting hundreds of FM patients with their disability claims over the years, I can honestly say that the process can be brutal, arduous and, oftentimes, downright demeaning for these patients. Many lose their homes and all financial security. Some lose their families and all other means of social and emotional support. I've even seen some patients lose their doctors over this.

The third counter-argument, which now shall be discussed in greater detail, is that FM exists everywhere, even in places and in populations where there is virtually no insurance to help the invalid, nor compensation to assist the injured. In fact, in some instances, it is more common in populations with little to no disability coverage than in those that are much more richly serviced.

Lest there be any confusion, FM and chronic, widespread pain both are common in wealthy, more industrialized countries too, where they exert considerable social and economic burdens(116). For example, two large North American studies placed the overall prevalence of FM in non-institutionalized adults (e.g., not in hospital or a group home) as being between 2.0% and 3.3%(13;117). These two studies also found FM to be more common in women than men (3.4% versus 0.5% in Wichita, Kansas; 4.9% versus 1.6% in London, Ontario). And, because of the relatively large number of female FM cases we confirmed in our London study, we were able to say with 95% confidence that FM prevalence increases as women age, peaking near 10% in those between the ages of 55 and 64, before steadily declining; in other words, roughly one in ten non-institutionalized women between the ages of 55 and 64 years old and living in London Ontario were found to have FM. Males exhibited a similar age-prevalence curve, peaking at 1.6%; but the fact that we confirmed significantly fewer male cases made our estimates by age group less reliable. For a sense of perspective, however, let's look at those peak prevalence figures. That almost 10% of women and 1.6% of men had FM in late middle-age implies that AT LEAST one in ten women and one in just over 60 men will develop FM at some point in their life. Suppose, then, that you are attending a sporting event at an outdoor stadium seating 50,000 people, half women and half men. What this means is that, as your eyes scan the crowd, you will be looking at roughly

2,500 women and 400 men who either have or will have FM at some point. Such numbers are staggering.

Fibromyalgia also is common throughout the more affluent countries of Western (versus Eastern) Europe, generally affecting between 0.5% and 2.5% of the general population(118-127), again with prevalence rates higher in women than men, reaching as high as 10% in women living in one Norwegian community(128).

However, FM also has been proven common in countries outside North America and Western Europe, like Mexico(129-131), Brazil(132;133), Poland(118), Turkey(134), Israel(17;135;136), Saudi Arabia(137), South Africa(138), Pakistan(139), Bangladesh(140), Malaysia(141), Thailand(142), Indonesia(143), and Japan(144). These populations span the globe and are tremendously diverse, both racially and culturally. Hence, the critic-insinuated stereotype of the lazy Westerner who has read about FM in a magazine and now decides to try it out to garner sympathy, an easier life, or both, clearly does not hold. In several instances, the prevalence of FM has been found to be higher in less affluent countries -- for example, in Pakistan(139), Bangladesh(140), Poland(118), and South Africa(138) -- than in countries in which the availability of disability insurance and compensation for injuries should be greater, like Sweden(119), Denmark(122), and Finland(121). In fact, the highest reported general population prevalence rates of FM have been 4.5% in Poland(118) and 4.4% in both Brazil(132) and Bangladesh(140), these three estimates all more than twice the 2.0% prevalence identified in Wolfe's U.S. study(117). Also, interestingly, the poorest, largely uninsured (in terms of disability insurance) segment of the Brazilian population(132) seems to be at greater risk for FM than those in Brazil who are more affluent(133).

One exception to the common worldwide prevalence of FM appears to be China, where FM only was found in about one person per 2000(145). However, the methods used to collect the initial data are not readily available, so there may have been flaws in study design, not uncommon to studies in poorer countries. In addition, rheumatoid arthritis appears to be equally rare in China, with a prevalence of just 0.2% to 0.3%, considerably lower than the roughly 1% reported almost anywhere else; and no one is suggesting that RA is not real? Finally, as Felson states:

"... the absence of fibromyalgia in China could be explained by genetic differences in the processing of afferent nociceptors throughout the body or by the absence of central sensitization, a phenomenon thought to be closely tied to the development of fibromyalgia. Clearly some causes of fibromyalgia are sociocultural, and it is possible that the different cultural environment in China might affect the acceptability of reporting chronic generalized pain.(146)"

In other words, the low rate of FM found in China may have been related to flaws in study design, to genetic differences in the Chinese versus other populations so that they have a reduced risk of FM, and/or to the Chinese being reluctant to admit to having widespread pain even when they have it.

So... is FM merely caused by over-generous disability insurance and compensation systems? It's hard to justify such a conclusion based upon the condition's high prevalence in Bangladesh, Pakistan, Poland, and the slums of Rio de Janeiro where few, if any, would have access to the 'generous' compensation systems available in the West.

CHAPTER 6: REASON #3
IT AFFECTS ALL POPULATIONS

In Chapter 5, I revealed how FM is everywhere, not just in rich, industrialized, Western nations with generous compensation systems. Again, where FM appears to be the most common is in places like Poland(118), Brazil(132), Pakistan(139), and Bangladesh(140), hardly countries with money to hand out to people 'faking' illness or disability. But, even in the West, FM affects people you would not expect, if FM is truly a compensation-driven illness, as some have claimed(76;111;112).

Two particularly intriguing populations in which fibromyalgia occurs are children(17;131) and the Amish(147).

Fibromyalgia in Children

Juvenile fibromyalgia is now a well-characterized syndrome, having become increasingly recognized and accepted over the past two decades(17;131;136;148-182) since publication of the 1990 American College of Rheumatology (ACR) criteria for FM; though it had been suspected and described previously(183;184). Like FM in adults, it is diagnosed using the 1990 ACR criteria of chronic, widespread pain, plus localized tenderness at no fewer than 11 of 18 specified anatomic points on the body (tender points)(81). As in adults, it is distributed widely, and in both industrialized countries - like Canada(180); the U.S.(157;167;170;177); those of Western Europe (e.g., Germany(156), Italy(175;179), and Iceland(155)); Scandinavia (Finland(168;171) and Sweden(176)); and Israel(17;148;178); and in less industrialized countries like Mexico(131), Brazil(174) and Turkey(185). In general-population surveys of school age children, its prevalence has ranged from just over one percent to as high as 7.5 percent(131;167;171;175;178). As in adults, females outnumber males by at least a two

61

to one margin in virtually all studies. And it seems to be relatively common both in children above and below the age of 10, with tremendous similarities in disease expression in these two age groups(157).

The clinical picture is very similar from location to location and country to country, and very much how it appears in adults, with poor sleep, fatigue, headaches, and muscle stiffness the most common symptoms, all reported by a majority(151;155;157;164;167;170;182-184). Many are quite disabled by their symptoms, resulting in problems at home, at school, and with their peers(152;158;161;163). The course, however, appears to be better in the young, though a sizeable percentage continue to have widespread pain and disability, as well as other symptoms. In a study by Gedalia and associates in New Orleans, for example, when reassessed an average of 18 months after initially being seen and diagnosed with FM, 30 of 50 patients (60%) were improved, but 20 (40%) were either the same or worse, and 27 (74%) still were taking medications for their FM(167). In Finland, the picture among 132 pre-adolescents and 16 adolescents was somewhat rosier, with only 30% and 25% still meeting the criteria for FM one year later, but significant symptoms and disability persisted in that sizable minority (168;171). Lest anyone suggest that the better outlook in the young versus old indicates that the FM in youths isn't real, note that the same favourable outlook in children and adolescents is true of many well-established and universally-accepted diseases, like leukaemia(186); and I believe that not one of these FM critics would suggest that leukaemia doesn't exist.

As for objective findings of disease, sleep studies show much the same abnormalities in children and adolescents as in adults(166;174;187), including the alpha wave intrusion into deep sleep that will be described in greater detail in a later chapter (Chapter 10), thereby demonstrating measurable dysfunction that could not possibly be manipulated by the children. And, though depression, anxiety, and other symptoms of psychological distress are common, when psychological status has been examined, symptoms of psychological distress are no more common than in other children and adolescents with comparable degrees of pain from other causes like rheumatoid arthritis(161;172).

Fibromyalgia in the Amish

Compared to a relative wealth of research on FM in children, there is very little studying this disorder in religiously-cloistered populations like the Amish. This is not surprising, because such populations often shun participation in Western style research. One study that does stand out is our own here in south-western Ontario(147). The results from this study are particularly intriguing because the Amish categorically refuse all government intervention, including any insurance or compensation coverage. And yet, FM was found to be more common in an Amish population in Ontario than in non-Amish(147), with prevalence rates of 7.3% and 3.2%, respectively. These Amish individuals reported the same widespread pain, disabling fatigue, and other symptoms as FM sufferers in other populations, and many reported significant disabilities in their daily activities.

Like all the studies that have found FM to be common in non-Western developing countries, and those finding it in children, the Amish study results form a strong argument against FM being compensation-driven, as some authors have claimed(111;112). Why would children and the Amish, and those living in Bangladesh, arguably the poorest country in the world, "choose to be a patient with chronic widespread pain", as one author contends(77)? The likely answer is: they wouldn't. People don't choose to have FM.

Given this, why do some critics continue to claim that FM is just a clever ploy for the lazy to get rich? Maybe it is because such FM critics fear it, much in the way some fear the fictitious Snark.

What is a Snark? Christopher Eccleston, a British researcher and author, refers to research on chronic, widespread pain in children as "Hunting the Snark", referring to the ferocious, fictitious animal that Lewis Carroll wrote about in his nonsense poem *The Hunting of the Snark*. Eccleston does not question the existence of the pain, nor its legitimacy or significance. Instead, he implores researchers to "do all that you know, and try all that you don't"(153). That is what so many current and past FM researchers,

63

like myself, have been doing... trying everything we can to get a grip on what is happening in so many people, of all ages, that is causing them so much pain, fatigue, other symptoms, disability and distress. In my opinion, many vocal FM critics, who do nothing but criticize the research of others without doing research themselves, fear such research, because proving the legitimacy of disorders like FM can only hinder their own agendas, whatever they may be.

CHAPTER 7: REASON #4
STRIKING SIMILARITIES EXIST
FROM PERSON TO PERSON

Let's assume, for a moment, that FM truly isn't real; that everyone with FM is either just depressed, or emotionally stressed, or exaggerating, or downright faking it. Critics have claimed all of these things.

Let's also assume, given an average prevalence of FM of between 2 and 4 percent in women and between 0.5 and 1.0 percent in men, that all these people learned about FM from the internet or books or by word of mouth. First of all, given that it has been reported not uncommonly in children, in North America alone, this would amount to about 5-6 million people, and roughly 100 million worldwide. How likely is it that all these individuals would be able to report the same symptoms... the widespread pain, hurting everywhere; not necessarily difficulty sleeping, but poor sleep, such that they feel tired no matter how long they sleep; the profound fatigue, both mental and physical; the stiffness; the worsening with activity but little to no relief with rest; and the generalized body tenderness? I suggest that such universal synchronization of symptoms is not very likely, if the condition truly is some sort of mass hysteria. But the fact is that the vast majority of FM patients, around the world, report the same constellation of major symptoms, and have done so since the syndrome initially was described back in the 1970s(14;15;28;108;188-196).

When individuals with FM are identified through a general population survey (for example, by being randomly selected for telephone screening interviews), as opposed to being recruited from a physician's practice or a subspecialty clinic, they again demonstrate the same constellation of major symptoms as those reported in clinic studies(117;197-199), making the possibility of 'learned' symptoms less likely: what possible incentive would people not seeking health services or some sort of disability coverage have to learn about FM and then fake it? In our own general population survey of adults living in London Ontario, out of the 100 cases of FM we confirmed, only about one third admitted to having heard about FM(92).

In addition to the traditional, major symptoms of FM, other very common and highly problematic symptoms are weakness, explained as difficulty holding an object for a period of time, rather than lifting it initially (a problem of muscle endurance or fatiguing versus true weakness); dizziness; difficulties with memory and concentration; irritability; cold sensitivity and numbness in hands and skin discolouration in cold weather (a characteristic called *Raynaud's phenomenon*); urinary frequency (having to urinate more often than normal, often with some discomfort while passing urine); and headaches(92). Some of these symptoms follow from general descriptions of FM; but others do not. In what commonly available literature, for example, would anyone read about the difference between muscle weakness and muscle fatigue; or about Raynaud's phenomenon; or about urinary frequency as a common FM complaint; or about dizziness? In other words, several less intuitive symptoms of FM are reported not uncommonly among patients seen in the clinic or cases of FM identified in population surveys, but are not mentioned in public literature, so that it is not likely that they are 'learned'.

Also, males and females do not differ in the range or nature of symptoms reported, other than women generally reporting more symptoms being a major problem for them over the preceding two weeks (9 versus 6) than men(92). But those who meet the diagnostic criteria for FM (having chronic widespread pain and at least 11 FM tender points) do differ, statistically, in numerous ways from those who either have chronic localized pain or chronic widespread pain but fewer than 11 tender points(92). For example, they are statistically more likely to report muscle fatigue; severe fatigue lasting 24 hours after minimal exertion; severe pain; glandular swelling in their neck; and overall poor health(92), some of which follows from published descriptions of FM and some of which does not.

What this means is that, if FM in fact IS all some big hoax, with some instruction manual out there that would-be fakers can read, that manual must be (1) extremely well hidden from doctors and researchers of FM, and from insurers and their lawyers, and from FM critics; but (2) ridiculously simple for everyone else to find.

Again, this isn't at all likely.

CHAPTER 8: REASON #5
IT'S NOT JUST A PROBLEM OF TAUTOLOGY

It was Cohen and Quintner who first detailed the so-called *tautological problem* associated with fibromyalgia(200), but many subsequent critics have fallen back upon this argument to justify their anti-FM stances.

What does the word *tautology* mean? If you Google the word, Wikipedia is the first reference; and it gives you this:

> Tautology (rhetoric): repetition of meaning, using different words to say the same thing twice, especially where the additional words fail to provide additional clarity when repeating a meaning.

Another way to think of it is as circular logic; and a good example of circular logic is something a student might say: "There's no way I deserve a 'B' in this class, because I only get 'A's." An even more blatant example is: "That can't be wrong, because it's right."

The tautological argument against fibromyalgia is that it only exists because a number of doctors got together and said it exists. To review from an earlier chapter, this is how the list of criteria we currently use to define FM came into being. A committee of physician researchers interested in studying certain patients they'd seen with widespread pain got together to define better what previously had been called *fibrositis* or *fibromyalgia* (FM)(81). They drew up a list of possible symptoms and physical findings (to find on examination) they thought would distinguish people with versus those without FM. They then studied 265 of their own patients, drawn from centers all across the U.S. and Canada, who they previously had diagnosed with FM, and compared them with a similar number of their patients who they felt did not have FM. And they found that the characteristics of (1) widespread pain (which they defined in a

69

particular way – see Chapter 2); (2) continuous pain lasting at least three months; and (3) tenderness at no fewer than 11 of 18 anatomically fixed body sites, were able to distinguish the 265 pre-conceived to have FM from those not pre-conceived to have FM.

But what if they had been wrong in the first place? What if many among the 265 who they previously had diagnosed with FM didn't REALLY have it? Maybe they had other, yet undiagnosed things; or maybe they had nothing really at all. And what if some of those whom the doctors didn't think have FM actually did? In other words, the doctors had decided beforehand what FM looked like, so drawing up a short list (with just a few criteria on it) to justify their preconceived notions makes no sense. At first glance, it seems akin to saying: "It's blue because we say it's blue."

But here's the rub against this tautological argument: how else would the critics have them do it? Given that there is no *gold standard*, universally reliable test (like a blood test or X-ray) that proves someone has FM, how could anyone know beforehand who really had FM and who really didn't? And, if there was such a test, why would anyone bother to come up with criteria in the first place? Just do the gold standard test.

The fact is that **there are many other well-accepted medical conditions that use criteria that were designed using exactly the same methods that were used for FM.** There is no gold standard test for rheumatoid arthritis (RA); or for systemic lupus erythematosus (lupus, SLE); or for a number of other diseases. For RA(201) and SLE(202), for example, classification criteria exist that were established using the same exact circular methodology as for FM, and that are little more sensitive (able to identify those with the condition) or specific (able to identify those who don't have the condition) than the 1990 FM criteria. Many other conditions have similarly generated criteria. Currently, for example, there is a large focus group of experts working to establish classification criteria for the poorly understood but very much accepted condition called polymyalgia rheumatica (PMR)(203). So, I ask, why do the FM critics appear to have no problem accepting the ways in which RA and SLE are defined? The answer is, I believe, either ignorance of these other criteria, or some personal agenda such that they don't want to look at other conditions. Either way, the tautological argument is shot down.

But what, some critics ask, about the person who has chronic widespread pain and fatigue and several other symptoms suggestive of FM, but only 10 tender points? Don't they have FM too? In all likelihood, they do. Note that the criteria for RA, SLE and every other condition for which such criteria exist also fail sometimes. In fact, even gold standard' tests are wrong sometimes. As evidence of this, I mention the case of a nurse I have known who was diagnosed with a rare and almost always fatal form of leukaemia. Rather than go through chemotherapy and feel sick all the time, with little chance for recovery, she decided to die on a beach in Hawaii, so as to enjoy the last few months the doctors told her she had left. Several years later, she returned from Hawaii with a clean bill of health, not having ever been treated for leukaemia. Did her cancer just go away, on its own? It's possible. But more likely the original tests were wrong.

Every diagnostic test that has been developed has a certain level of sensitivity and specificity ascribed to it, determined by research to identify how often the test is right, and how often it's wrong. No test is right all the time. So, back to FM... what about the person with chronic widespread pain and 10 tender points? They are no more of a problem than the person who seems to have SLE but only meets 3 of 11 criteria, or the person who seems to have RA but has only 3 of 7 criteria. Probably, these patients have SLE and RA, respectively, just like the person with chronic widespread pain but only 10 of 18 tender points probably has FM. Similarly, the patient with localized pain and more than 11 tender points likely has some other pain condition, like *myofascial pain*(204); though some of these individuals may progress to full FM over time, and some might meet the ACR's most recent preliminary diagnostic criteria(83) even with only localized pain, if they have certain other severe symptoms (like fatigue and waking up non-rested) as well.

71

The fact is that **we are led to believe that there are 999 diseases; but this is false. In truth, there are 999 disease labels.** Some of these labels work well. For example, the diabetes label generally is a good one, because glucose testing is inexpensive, and easily repeated, and enough patients with high blood sugars have been followed in studies long enough for doctors and others to know that leaving chronically elevated blood sugars alone for too long is a bad thing. The fibromyalgia label is not so good a label; but neither is the rheumatoid arthritis label; or the lupus label; or the PMR label (I will be bringing PMR up again in a later chapter, because it will help me to demonstrate flaws in other anti-FM arguments); or the migraine headache label. In fact, as aptly illustrated by Harth and Nielson(84), one of the worst labels is for high blood pressure, because the vast majority of people who meet the criteria for high blood pressure (also called *hypertension*) never experience symptoms or problems from it, other than perhaps side effects from their medications to control it; and sometimes, persons with normal blood pressure suffer consequences typically ascribed to hypertension (like strokes and heart attacks). This latter concern has prompted the Joint National Committee on Prevention, Detection, Evaluation and Treatment of High Blood Pressure to define blood pressures from 120/80 to 139/89 as *pre-hypertension*(205).

As a final example, let's look away from medicine towards nature. What is a hurricane, what is a typhoon, and what is a cyclone? No doubt there are specific definitions for each of these, and considerable debate among experts as to how to define each. But, to the person whose house has just blown down, does any of this matter? Until there is a gold standard diagnostic test for FM, debate will rage as to what the term means or should mean, and when or if it should be used. But to say that the label is any worse than the labels for many other well-accepted conditions for which the same scientific methods were used is grossly unfair. Many a person with FM has felt the world that they knew, before they became sick, totally blown apart. Shouldn't that be enough to warrant at least a little bit of compassion and help from the rest of us?

CHAPTER 9: REASON #6

NUMEROUS BIOCHEMICAL ABNORMALITIES HAVE BEEN REPORTED

Another popular argument used by fibromyalgia critics is that there's just no evidence of disease. One author described it as being the same old aches and pains that everyone has(76;77). It's just that some people cope better than others.

If this is true -- if, in fact, people with FM are no different than anyone else -- then they should be no different from 'normal' whenever you do various blood and urine and other tests on them. And, in fact, they typically are not different, in terms of the tests doctors routinely order in their offices. Patients with FM appear to be no more likely to have low or high blood counts, sodium or potassium levels, etc., than people without FM.

Case closed? Hardly! And I say this for two reasons. **First, there are many other well-accepted disorders for which routine blood and urine tests and X-rays typically fall within the range of normal** ... autism and schizophrenia come to mind first, but some may claim these are 'mental diseases'. But what about migraines? What about headaches in general? What about shingles AFTER the rash has disappeared? Shingles patients can have excruciating chronic pain, sometimes for years, long after the rash is gone and in the absence of ANY routine lab or imaging abnormalities (by imaging, I refer to X-rays, but also CAT scans and MRIs). What about an excruciatingly painful nerve condition called *trigeminal neuralgia*[§]? What about *phantom limb pain*? As described in the next chapter, there is fairly conclusive evidence that phantom limb pain really exists: among other things, rats get it, and what hidden agenda could rats possibly have? But more about this later.

[§] The term *neuralgia* means nerve pain; and the trigeminal nerve is a nerve that provides sensation to the face.

My first point is that there are many well-accepted diseases for which routine labs and imaging show nothing at all.

And my second point is that **FM patients DO, in fact, have biochemical and physiological and other abnormalities; just not among the tests doctors <u>routinely</u> order.** The next chapter will expand on abnormalities that probably are behind why persons with FM feel like they do. This chapter won't go that far. Here, I'll merely list and briefly describe some of the numerous (and I do mean numerous) abnormalities that have been scientifically demonstrated to be significantly more common in FM patients than in persons without FM. These abnormalities can be found in the blood, in spinal fluid, in the way blood flows, in the way skin reacts, and in the nerves and brain. I don't need to list every single one to prove my point; but here are several examples. It is important to note that all of these findings have been discovered despite the fact that fibromyalgia tends to receive far less research funding support than other diseases like lupus, rheumatoid arthritis and osteoporosis(206):

- Alterations in chemicals called *neurotransmitters*[**], including elevated spinal fluid levels of **pain agonists** (that are released by nerves to transmit the perception of pain to the brain), like substance P(73;74;207-209); and decreased spinal fluid and blood levels of **pain antagonists** (that are released by nerves to reduce the perception of pain in the brain), like serotonin and related chemicals(193;210-217). Substance P also has been found to be elevated in the muscles of women with FM and those with localized myofascial pain, relative to the levels found in healthy women(218).

- Alterations in tissue blood flow, including inadequate blood flow to muscles in response to muscle use(219;220); altered levels of blood flow (often decreased)

[**] Neurotransmitters help to transmit nerve impulses along nerve pathways. In a crude way, a neurotransmitter is to a nerve what a train is to a train track.

to certain parts of the brain(207;221-225;225-228); and deviations from normal in cerebral (brain) blood flow in response to various painful and non-painful stimuli, like warmth, light touch, pressure delivered via compressed air, and speech(229-236). Moreover, these deviations from normal seem to negatively correlate with immune activity within the brain; as flow decreases, some aspects of immune activity increase. This suggests a possible role of the immune system in FM, which may explain why FM is more common in autoimmune diseases like lupus and rheumatoid arthritis(237).

• Altered sleep, including disordered brain waves in deep sleep that, interestingly, correlate with the patient's degree of pain(107;187;238;239); in other words, the more disrupted their sleep brain waves are, the more pain they have.

• Other abnormalities in the way the brain processes information, like its processing of sound(231;232;240-242), which may relate to why FM patients have difficulty concentrating and remembering things; and its processing of other non-painful external stimuli, like cold and light touch, that may contribute to some of the other manifestations of this disease.

• Hormonal changes, including abnormal through-the-day fluctuations in serum levels of cortisol(243), reduced morning levels of cortisol that correlate with the degree of morning symptoms(244), a two to three-fold increase in risk of FM among persons who are deficient in thyroid hormone (hypothyroid)(42), a 15-fold increased risk of FM among persons who have elevated blood levels of a hormone called prolactin(245), and low serum levels of somatomedin-C(246), growth hormone(247), and a hormone that is critical in the repair of injured muscles, called *insulin-like growth factor*(248;249).

• Alterations in the autonomic (involuntary) nervous system that, as opposed to nerves that give us sensation and motor control, controls such things as our blood pressure, heart rate, and skin temperature. The autonomic nervous system

75

controls skin temperature by regulating the flow of blood to the skin. The various autonomic nervous system irregularities that are seen in FM patients but not in those without it include: skin temperature that is reduced in the back(250) but higher in the hands(251) in FM patients versus healthy controls; prolonged sympathetic responses in the skin of the palm and sole when the median and tibial nerves in the opposite limb (e.g., right arm stimulated; left arm tested) are electrically stimulated(252); orthostatic hypotension, which is disrupted control of blood pressure when someone goes from lying to standing(253), the normal adjustments made in blood vessel muscle tone lacking in FM patients (which may explain some of their dizziness); and a phenomenon called *reactive hyperaemia*, which is exaggerated blood flow to the skin in response to transient pain (like pinching or a pin prick)(254;255).

- Increased levels of a critical chemical called *brain-derived neurotrophic factor* (BDNF), a protein involved in nerve survival and the plasticity of nerve synapses within the central and peripheral nervous system(256). In addition, BDNF serum concentrations were independent of the patient's age, gender, length of illness, pre-existing recurrent major depression, and the use of anti-depressant medications in low doses, suggesting that BDNF might be involved in the pathophysiology of pain in FM, rather than an indicator of something else like depression.

- Structural abnormalities in the brain, with increased and decreased volumes of grey matter in different brain regions(257), with similar abnormalities also detectable in patients with chronic headaches and chronic back pain(258;259).

- Abnormal levels of various indicators of energy and muscle repair in muscles, including adenosine triphosphate (ATP), the main energy transfer and storage molecule in cells, both during rest and during exercise, all detectable using an advanced imaging technique called *magnetic resonance spectroscopy* (MRS)(260). Note that MRS is similar to magnetic resonance imaging (MRI); but it looks at levels of specific atomic particles (in this case, phosphate P-31) instead of generating pictures like MRI. The abnormally low levels of ATP in the muscles of FM patients are consistent with the fatigue and muscle weakness reported by patients.

- Myofascial trigger points not found in healthy individuals that exhibit a local 'twitch response' when poked with a needle, demonstrate spontaneous, abnormal electrical activity on electromyelogram (EMG), and appear abnormal when imaged by 2-dimensional ultrasound(261-263).

- Microscopic abnormalities in small blood vessels under the nails(264;265).

- A genetic predisposition, with clustering of cases within families and evidence of a specific type of chromosomal defect affecting serotonin-related and catecholamine-related pain pathways, particularly affecting an enzyme called *catecholamine-O-methyltransferase* (COMT), similar to one that is observed in those with temperomandibular (jaw) joint (TMJ) pain(148;266-270).

- And the list goes on and on.

Clearly then, the contention that those with FM are no different than anyone else other than being chronic complainers is false. They are different, in numerous ways that could not possibly be manipulated for purposes of deceiving others, or just being lazy.

Anti-FM critics may argue that there have been inconsistencies in these laboratory results, as there have been. For example, whereas Leal-Cerro and associates found spontaneous growth hormone release to be reduced(247), Denko and Malemud found baseline growth hormone levels to be elevated(271). Having said this, hormone levels always fluctuate widely in response to different situations and times of the day; so it may not be the absolute level of these hormones that is important, but how they rise or fall in different situations and at different times.

Moreover, most of the abnormalities that have been identified in FM patients have been remarkably consistent from study to study and from place to place, and at least as consistent as in most other diseases. For example, many of the treatments that doctors prescribe for a variety of illnesses, though proven effective in some studies, have not been proven effective in others. In most instances, the weight of evidence favours the particular treatment's efficacy, and that is why physicians prescribe it. But there still were negative studies. Should we stop using a particular drug because one out of 11 studies that were done found it to be ineffective? Of course not. Experiments fail for a large number of reasons that I won't go into here. That is why they must be repeated, as they have been for fibromyalgia. And the overwhelming number of studies have identified FM patients as being physiologically different than those who are healthy, and those with other disease states.

Critics also may say that some of these physiological abnormalities are secondary to such things as muscle de-conditioning, and certainly that might be true of some of the muscle changes(272;273) and the drop in blood pressure some patients experience upon standing. But muscle de-conditioning, in itself, does not at all preclude some other underlying cause of disease. In fact, such de-conditioning is observed in most chronically ill individuals(274).

Others say that these abnormalities are manifestations of depression or anxiety, and perhaps a few of them are. But such arguments cannot possibly explain all of these abnormal findings. How, for example, would depression or anxiety explain reactive hyperaemia, or the low levels of growth hormone?

Moreover, as I will discuss again in a later chapter (Chapter 15), depression is now known to be a biochemically-based disease too. So saying someone isn't sick because

78

they are depressed makes no sense at all. "Yes you have cancer. But you also are depressed, so we see no need to treat your cancer!" Could you imagine a doctor actually saying that?

Tragically, what many anti-FM critics continuously espouse is the same kind of grossly flawed and uncaring logic.

CHAPTER 10 - REASON #7

SCIENTIFICALLY-SUPPORTED AND LOGICAL

EXPLANATIONS EXIST

In the last chapter, I described numerous abnormalities that are found in patients with fibromyalgia to a greater extent than in people without fibromyalgia. More of these abnormalities exist; I only mentioned some of them.

But what actually causes FM? This question is important to the person who suffers from this condition; and I am sure it is of interest to many who care for them, either professionally as a health care provider, or personally as a family member or friend. But it also is crucial from a medicolegal standpoint, for two major reasons:

1.   Even a partial understanding of a condition's cause lends credence to its existence. The corollary to this is that, if there is no way you can hypothesize something coming into existence, how can it possibly exist? I call this the Big Bang versus Big Bust Theory of Illness.

        AND

2.   The issue of trauma as a cause of fibromyalgia is huge in the medicolegal setting, especially relating to whiplash and workplace injuries.

If you surf through the internet, you will come up with a thousand or more answers as to what causes FM; everything from ammonia excess to zinc deficiency. No one really knows with absolute certainty. But that is not the same as saying that we have no idea. As stated in the last chapter, there is a large body of scientific research that has shown numerous biochemical and physiological abnormalities in people with FM that distinguish them from those who are healthy and/or those with other medical conditions.

Several excellent scientific reviews have been written and published in high-profile scientific journals describing the probable mechanisms of disease in FM(209;217;275-280).

The objective of this chapter is not to go through them all again. However, there are four broad areas of abnormalities that almost certainly are critical in understanding the cause or causes of symptoms in FM. These broad areas are:

1. Neurotransmitter dysfunction
2. Sleep dysfunction
3. Altered blood flow to brain and muscles
4. Neuroplasticity

Terms like *neurotransmitter* and *neuroplasticity* will be defined in the following pages. But first, critical to understanding the relative roles of each of these four areas is some understanding of what pain is.

WHAT IS PAIN?

To begin with, pain is useful. Pain tells us to take our hand out of the fire. Pain tells us not to put our full weight down if we are stepping barefoot on broken glass. Pain tells us to seek help if we are bitten by a snake. Pain keeps us alive.

If we had no perception of pain, we would not live long. In fact, there was a young woman in Montreal who was born without the ability to feel pain(281). She did not live long. She died in her late twenties of pneumonia after having broken virtually every one of her ribs from coughing. She just didn't know when she was coughing too hard. She already had broken so many bones that she could barely walk and had premature arthritis. This patient was described in detail in a landmark book, called *The Challenge of Pain*, by leading pain researchers Melzack and Wall(281).

So... pain is useful. But prolonged pain is much less useful. You don't need to be an internationally-recognized expert in pain to realize that you don't put your hand in the fire twice. And so, **we have a system in our body by which pain is turned on... and pain is turned off.**

A good example of this happened to me several years ago. It was one of those rare days when I was home during a work day. My wife had driven our four kids to school and daycare. I had agreed to pick them up at the end of their day. I was upstairs in a bedroom, folding laundry, when I glanced at the clock and saw that it was 5:10 PM. I needed to leave right away, so as not to be late picking up our youngest from daycare by 5:25. Hence, I started two-stepping down the stairs to get to the front door and out to the car. Now, we have hardwood stairs that circle around a corner, so that the inner part of some stairs is very narrow at the turn. Unfortunately, my right foot missed the fourth stair from the top. Down I went, sliding down 15 stairs, all the way on my right side. By the time I hit the first floor, I was sure I'd broken my hip. I lay there in agony, wondering what to do. It only took me about 60 seconds to realize that it probably would hurt less if I rolled off of my injured hip. As I did so, I fully expected to hear my hip bone (femur) snap. But it did not. It then took me another minute or so to realize that I was still lying against the steps and that this was uncomfortable on my back. So I slowly sat up, again fully expecting my hip to snap into several pieces. And again, it did not. I very slowly and carefully tried to stand up on one leg so I could hop to the phone in the kitchen to call my wife to tell her to pick up the kids. Standing up took about two minutes. By this time, the pain in my hip was less that it had been, and the crazy thought was filling my brain that maybe, just maybe, my hip was not broken after all. Very gingerly, I placed a little bit of weight on my right foot. Nothing happened. A little more weight. Okay so far. Then I took a step. I limped around very carefully for about five more steps, and it dawned on me that my hip probably was not broken. It also dawned on me that the whole reason I'd been running down the stairs in the first place was that I was late going to pick up my kids. I hobbled out to the car and drove to get them. By the time I returned home 45 minutes later with my children, I was walking with almost no limp. I had minimal pain. But my hip was still extremely tender to touch. About one week later, I was getting out of the shower. My wife glanced over at me and nearly fainted (and she doesn't usually do that when she sees me). I looked down to see that I was virtually black all the way from my right hip down to my knee -- a huge black bruise.

So... how did I go from being sure I'd broken my hip, to thinking maybe I hadn't, to pretty sure I hadn't, to sure I hadn't, to no real pain at all but still tender, all within about an hour... to a huge black bruise that really didn't hurt at all one week later? I'd obviously hurt myself and the evidence of tissue damage was still there one week later.

The answer is: the pain on, pain off system that I've already mentioned, that virtually everybody has (except a very few documented cases).

The reality is that, although the FM patient has pain in muscles and fibrous tissues (according to the name), in fact the true disease in FM almost certainly is within the nervous system itself. Again, pain is useful, but normally there is a system that shuts pain down, or at least dampens it, within a few minutes to hours of whatever injury caused the pain in the first place. In FM, that pain on/pain off system is dysfunctional.

Neurotransmitter Dysfunction

There are a large number of chemicals within the nervous system that are important to the pain on, pain off system. They belong to a class of chemicals called *neurotransmitters*. Using a somewhat inaccurate but still useful analogy, neurotransmitters are to a nerve, what a train is to a train track. Just like trains 'transmit' new cars down the line between Detroit and Toronto, neurotransmitters transmit messages along nerve pathways and between nerves so that the pain of a bee sting reaches our spinal cord and our brain. In our nervous system, we have neurotransmitters that activate or augment pain perception, called *pain agonists*. These chemicals are released by our nerves immediately after a painful event, like a bee sting. One important pain agonist is called *substance P*. We also have neurotransmitters that diminish our perception of pain, called *pain antagonists* (they antagonize or counteract the effects of chemicals like substance P). One important pain antagonist we have is called *serotonin*. Published research studies have consistently shown that people with FM have way too much substance P(73;74;207;208). Others have shown that FM patients have too little of the pain antagonist serotonin and its analogues(193;210-217). In other words, they have too much pain agonist, and not enough pain antagonist.

How might this affect the FM patient? Normally, if someone squeezes your hand, perhaps in greeting, there is no or minimal pain caused by that. If that person squeezes your hand too tightly, or for too long, it may become uncomfortable for you. Ultimately, you will want them to let go. Once they do let go, whatever discomfort the handshake may have caused dissipates within seconds. Among other things, the pain antagonist serotonin has come to the rescue to shut the pain off. However, what if the person whose hand was being squeezed has way too much substance P? What should happen? Answer: a heightened pain response. Even a relatively gentle squeeze may hurt, even right away. Then, after the handshake has ended, if they have too little serotonin (and other pain antagonists), the pain from the handshake may persist. Half an hour later, their hand still may hurt.

That is likely why many FM patients report that they cannot wash their hair. Normally, when someone washes their hair, holding their arms up to scrub their scalp causes mild muscle fatigue and minimal discomfort that goes away as soon as they put their arms back down again. A little substance P was released when their arms were up; but serotonin kicked in as soon as they rested their arms. Hence, they experience minimal, short-lived discomfort. Likely, among FM patients, too much substance P already is present and/or is released while their arms are up, so washing their hair actually hurts. Then, there is not enough serotonin and other antagonists around when they put their arms down; consequently, their arms may hurt for hours afterwards. After washing their hair, they may be done for the day.

Other neurotransmitters besides substance P and serotonin appear to be dysregulated in FM. In one, most interesting recent study, for example, spinal fluid levels of an opioid peptide (a normal neurotransmitter chemically similar to the narcotic pain-killer opium) called *met-enkephalin-Arg6-Phe7* (MEAP), were found to be elevated, both in patients with FM and those with back pain, relative to healthy individuals without pain(282). And perhaps most important of all is that a particular nerve receptor, called the *N-methyl-D-aspartic acid (NMDA) receptor*, which is found in the dorsal horn of the spinal cord, where sensory input from the body, like pain, is first transmitted to the spine, seems to act abnormally in persons with FM. The NMDA receptor plays a role in what has been called pain *wind up*, whereby after an initial painful stimulus, subsequent equal stimuli are felt to be even more painful. These receptors are normally inactive; but, with repeated stimulation, they turn on. In recent studies, NMDA hyper-excitability and the ability to reduce that hyper-excitability using an NMDA receptor antagonist, called *ketanserin*, have been demonstrated in FM patients(283;284).

More about Serotonin

As it turns out, serotonin is more than just a pain antagonist. It also is important in regulating blood flow to tissue. A synthetic form of serotonin, called *ketanserin* (please see the previous paragraph), has been used in the treatment of severely high blood pressure(285). It causes blood vessels to dilate (get bigger). Note that arteries are blood vessels that carry blood from our heart to the rest of our body. Every artery is a tube that is surrounded by a wall of muscle that contracts or relaxes to regulate the size of the blood vessel and, hence, the amount of blood travelling through that vessel. When the muscle contracts, the tube gets smaller, so less blood passes through. When the muscle relaxes, the tube gets bigger and more blood gets through. In FM, there is some evidence of inadequate blood flow to muscles in response to muscle use, though some researchers who have reported this failed to distinguish between patients with FM and those with myofascial pain syndrome (MPS). Such a shortage of blood flow, if it is a real manifestation of disease, undoubtedly could cause muscle fatigue, pain, and cramping. FM patients report all these things.

Also in FM, there is evidence of decreased blood flow to certain parts of the brain, and deviations from normal in cerebral (brain) blood flow, often associated with a regional increase in flow in response to various painful and non-painful stimuli, like warmth, light touch, pressure delivered via compressed air, and speech(229-236). Perhaps this explains at least some of the profound fatigue and mental fogginess that almost all FM patients experience (the term *fibro fog* has been coined). Consequently, the relative lack of serotonin also may induce pain, cramping, and muscle fatigue via deficient blood flow to muscles, and a variety of other symptoms via abnormal blood flow to the brain and other organs.

Finally, serotonin also seems to be very important in deep sleep which, as the next section will illustrate, is a major problem in FM.

What lends further credence to the importance of serotonin in FM is the fact that medications targeting serotonin receptors, specifically the receptor called 5-HT3, appear to have some beneficial effect(286). A serotonin deficiency can't be the entire story, however, because such medications tend to produce only modest reductions in pain and other symptoms.

Sleep Dysfunction

As stated in Chapter 1, sleep disturbance is an ever-present problem among FM patients. In our own study of 100 adults with FM identified through a survey of the general population, disordered sleep was reported by 92%; and disordered sleep was reported to be a major problem by two thirds(197). Among those with FM being seen by specialists for their FM, these figures are higher(3;15), probably because more severely affected individuals are more likely to be referred to a specialist.

The first research identifying the association between disrupted sleep and chronic pain was published in the 1970s by Moldofsky and Smythe in Toronto(104;105;108). Subsequent research has confirmed and expanded upon this association. To understand this better, it is necessary for you to understand the various stages of sleep.

There are five stages of sleep. Stage 1 is light sleep; Stage 2 a little deeper; Stage 3 deeper yet; and Stage 4 deeper yet. Rapid eye movement (REM) sleep is the stage of sleep in which we dream (and our sleeping dogs chase rabbits). These five different stages of sleep are distinguished by two different types of brain wave that can be detected if electrodes are placed on an individual's head to monitor for brain activity: alpha waves and delta waves. These two types of brain wave are depicted well in the following picture:

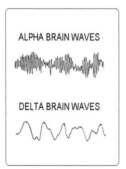

In Stage 1, virtually all the brain waves detected are high amplitude, rapid-firing alpha waves. Conversely, stage 4 sleep is characterized by a virtual absence of alpha waves, being filled with low amplitude, slow, rolling delta waves. Stages 2 and 3 are filled with a combination of the two types of brain wave, more alpha than delta in Stage 2 and more delta than alpha in Stage 3. Patients with FM are sorely deficient in stage 4 sleep.

Moldofsky has repeatedly tested FM patients over the years and found that they have dramatically diminished stage 4 (pure delta wave) sleep(239). The term *alpha wave intrusion* has been used to indicate that numerous alpha wave spikes are seen throughout what otherwise should be pure delta wave, stage 4 Sleep. More recently, Moldofsky and his research partners discovered that **the greater the number of alpha waves a person has in stage 4, the more pain and**

stiffness they have(107;187;238). **This is strong evidence that FM pain is real, since no one can possibly know or willingly influence how much alpha wave intrusion they have during sleep.**

In addition to an association between altered deep sleep and chronic pain, there is some evidence that such sleep disruption actually can <u>cause</u> widespread pain. About 30 years ago, Moldofsky and Scarisbrick induced chronic, widespread pain and profound fatigue in a group of previously-healthy medical students(106). Essentially, they placed electrodes on their heads and let them sleep. Then they provided a stimulus to knock them out of Stage 4 Sleep every time they entered into it. Within 72 hours, the students whose stage 4 sleep had been repeatedly interrupted hurt everywhere, were diffusely tender, and could barely stand up from fatigue. The good news for the students is that their pain went away after they were allowed to sleep normally again. Unfortunately, to date, no one has been able to return the altered sleep of FM patients to normal.

Adding to this is that chemical abnormalities associated with disrupted sleep also have been documented in persons with FM. Note foremost that substance P, which already has been mentioned as elevated in FM patients, is a known potent inhibitor of sleep(209). But other chemical abnormalities that have been documented by scientific research include deficiencies in nocturnal (night-time) levels of serotonin (as mentioned above), and the hormones cortisol(243), growth hormone(287;288), somatomedin-C (246), and melatonin(289). Moreover, injections of growth hormone have been shown to reduce the severity of FM symptoms in those patients previously found to be deficient(287). **All of this adds further credence both to FM as a legitimate disease, and to sleep disruption having some causative role.** The link between serotonin deficiencies and both the pain neurotransmitter imbalance and sleep disorder may prove especially important when all these causative mechanisms are clarified once and for all.

A few further words on Fibro Fog

The title for this book, *Breaking Thru the Fibro Fog*, was chosen for many reasons. One of them is the tremendous impact that this mental cloudiness or slowed thinking has upon so many with FM. Some patients say that they can deal with the pain and the fatigue; it's their inability to think clearly that they find most difficult to live with.

Some attribute fibro fog to the medications that many patients take for pain or sleep. But fibro fog is present in patients on medications, and in those not on medications, so this symptom cannot be attributed just to the medications themselves. As pointed out earlier in this chapter, decreased blood flow to the brain may play a role, as may the just-described profound fatigue, sleeplessness and poor quality sleep most FM patients must endure. Who among any of us, healthy or not, is at his or her best after staying up all night? Replace this one all-nighter with thousands of horrible sleeps, and it is no wonder that mental fogginess has become one of the most recognized symptoms of this condition.

But actual brain atrophy, which has been documented in FM, may be another factor contributing to this oftentimes debilitating facet of fibro.

Altered Blood Flow to Brain and Muscles

Several studies have demonstrated that there are abnormal alterations in the amount of blood that flows to various tissues in patients with FM. One that makes immediate sense is inadequate blood flow to muscles in response to muscle use(219;220), since muscles that are deprived of adequate blood flow experience cramping and pain. The cramps that runners get probably are related to this. So are heart attacks and angina, since the heart is, after all, a muscle.

Several studies also have demonstrated that, compared to healthy individuals and, sometimes, patients with other conditions, those with FM have decreased blood flow to certain parts of their brain(207;221-226) and abnormal cerebral (brain) blood flow responses, often associated with increased regional flow, when the patient is exposed to various painful and non-painful stimuli (229-236). This also makes sense, if we accept the overwhelming body of scientific evidence that FM is a disorder of the central nervous system primarily, and not just a muscle disease (or a muscle disease at all). Interestingly, one specific area of the brain that has been scientifically shown to be different, both in patients with FM and patients with chronic low back pain versus controls, is the hippocampus(290), which happens to be an area of the brain responsible for sleep regulation, pain perception, and several different cognitive functions. Not only that, but there is a well-described and widely-accepted condition called *thalamic syndrome* that often occurs in individuals who have suffered a stroke involving a part of the mid brain called the *thalamus*(291-297). What do these patients experience? In addition to problems with concentration and short-term memory, they typically have severe, generalized burning pain and tenderness involving the entire side of the body opposite the stroke (e.g., if the stroke involved the left thalamus, the pain and tenderness is on the patient's right side). Alterations in blood flow to the thalamus and adjacent areas of the brain also appear to be abnormal in familial cases of *restless leg syndrome*, a condition especially associated with night-time leg pain, and not at all uncommon in patients with FM(298).

The Neuroplasticity Concept

Neuroplasticity is a term that refers to the ability of nerves to undergo permanent changes over time. In a healthy state, they are not supposed to. When a nerve is stimulated, it is supposed to change long enough to transmit the impulse (be it pain or cold or sight) down the line, and then revert back to its resting state. There is evidence in patients with chronic pain, however, that nerves sometimes change permanently. The most classic example of this is phantom limb pain(299). As will be explained in greater detail in Chapter 16, when the issue of post-traumatic FM is discussed, neuroplasticity is a scientifically-supported and logistically-reasonable explanation for the widespread pain FM patients feel in the absence of persistent, visible tissue damage or chronic inflammation. Interestingly, many of the neurotransmitter and hormonal imbalances already described in this chapter also come into play within the neuroplasticity concept.

As just stated, neuroplasticity will be discussed in much greater detail in a later chapter. Suffice it to say that, along with the various neurotransmitter imbalances, sleep disturbances, and alterations in blood flow patterns clearly demonstrated in FM patients, it serves as yet another viable explanation for the chronic pain of FM.

To Sum Up...

When these four different but related mechanisms are taken together, it is clear that the overwhelming belief among fibromyalgia researchers is that FM is a disease of the central nervous system. This conjecture is supported by the proven, albeit limited, effectiveness of the drug *pregabalin*, and by its subsequent approval by the U.S. Federal Drug Administration for use in fibromyalgia(300). Note especially that pregabalin is a drug also approved for the treatment of neuralgia (nerve pain) and seizures, and that it is NOT an anti-depressant. I mention that pregabalin is not an anti-depressant because of the claim, by many anti-FM critics, that FM is just a physical manifestation of depression (see Chapter 15 for more on this).

More specifically, what is now widely considered to be the underlying mechanism of disease in FM is some disruption in what has been called *central processing* within the brain and spinal cord(209;268;275-279;301-304). In a nutshell, theorists all come back to the pain/on-pain off system that I described at the start of this chapter, though terms like *centralized hypersensitivity, excessive spinal excitatory activity, reduced descending inhibitory pathways,* and *diminished pain down-regulation* are more often used.

The admittedly incomplete picture on the following page briefly summarizes all of this:

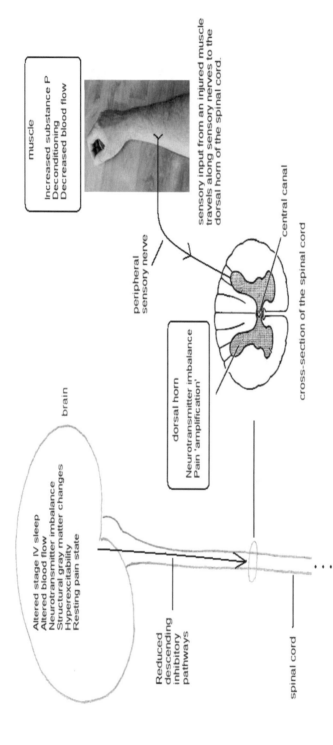

muscle

Increased substance P
Deconditioning
Decreased blood flow

sensory input from an injured muscle
travels along sensory nerves to the
dorsal horn of the spinal cord.

peripheral
sensory nerve

central canal

cross-section of the spinal cord

dorsal horn

Neurotransmitter imbalance
Pain 'amplification'

brain

Altered stage IV sleep
Altered blood flow
Neurotransmitter imbalance
Structural gray matter changes
Hyperexcitability
Resting pain state

Reduced
descending
inhibitory
pathways

spinal cord

Likely underlying disease pathways in fibromyalgia

Again, numerous excellently-written reviews theorizing about the mechanisms behind FM, given what is known scientifically, have been published. Of these, my personal favourite is one written by Harris and Clauw, called *How Do We Know That the Pain in Fibromyalgia Is 'Real'?* , that was published in *Current Pain and Headache Reports* in October 2006(268). Discussing FM primarily, but also other poorly-understood chronic pain disorders, the authors conclude by writing:

"It is time for us to move past the rhetoric about whether these conditions are real and take these patients seriously as we endeavour to learn more about the causes and most effective treatments for these disorders."

That truly is all that fibromyalgia critics are continuing to put forward... rhetoric... totally ignoring the huge body of evidence that exists demonstrating all the pathology that exists in FM. I think that it is long past time such rhetoric be laid to rest.

CHAPTER 11: REASON #8
THERE <u>ARE</u> OBJECTIVE FINDINGS

Some critics say that fibromyalgia doesn't exist because there are no physical findings; in other words, despite how they feel, these people look normal. They have no rash; no fever; no hot, swollen joints; no enlarged lymph nodes. Again, they LOOK normal. All patients with so-called *fibromyalgia* have is tenderness when the examiner pushes on them. And, worse than that, many are tender EVERYWHERE. Some doctors go so far as to rule FM out in a patient who is tender everywhere, because they are not just tender at the 18 points specified in the 1990 American College of Rheumatology (ACR) criteria for fibromyalgia. Doctors like this invariably test what they like to call *control points* (points other than the 18 criteria points), and say a person does not have FM if they are tender at these control points too.

Interestingly, many of these same physicians who have such difficulty understanding and accepting FM have no problems at all injecting or even operating upon patients with conditions like rotator cuff tendonitis (of the shoulder) or greater trochanteric bursitis (of the hip), despite the absence of 'objective' physical findings in many patients with either of these conditions.

There are three major counter-arguments against the "FM has no objective findings'" naysayers, and they are:

3. Tenderness is a widely-accepted indicator of underlying disease in countless other settings;

4. There are, actually, objective physical findings in many patients with FM, that are found more commonly than in people without FM; and

5. The use of *control points* to defrock FM makes no sense, given what we know about FM from extensive research.

Let's discuss each of these counter-arguments in sequence.

Tenderness is a widely-accepted physical sign in other settings

Last year, my youngest son, who is now 15-years old, woke up in the middle of the night with excruciating pain in his belly. The pain was so severe I had to carry him to the car; and this is a kid who completely shattered his thumb playing ice hockey and kept playing. In the emergency room of the hospital, he was examined thoroughly and repeatedly by the ER doctor. What concerned her most was not only the apparent severity of my son's pain, but also how exquisitely tender his abdomen was. She kept coming back to examine his belly for tenderness again and again. Otherwise, he had no fever. His heart rate was a bit fast, but no more than one would expect in someone complaining of pain, and within normal limits for some people. He had no rashes. His spleen and liver seemed to be of normal size. And even his labs came back normal; but still she kept coming back and examining him. What she was trying to decide was whether or not she should call a surgeon to explore the possibility of appendicitis. What eventually swayed her not to? Finally, after several hours, she decided to give my son a shot of morphine, and the pain relief was so immediate and dramatic, it convinced her that it couldn't be appendicitis, peritonitis or anything so serious. In fact, the final diagnosis was severe intestinal spasms; the morphine, because of its muscle relaxant qualities, had stopped the cramping, and therefore the pain. Luckily, this hasn't happened again.

But the points to be noted here are: *(1)* that the doctor believed my son's pain, in the absence of any physical finding other than extreme abdominal tenderness; and *(2)* that tenderness alone was valued by the doctor to the extent that she actually seriously considered calling a surgeon.

If you grab any medical school textbook describing how to perform a physical examination -- for example, Barbara Bates' *Guide to Physical Examination*(305) -- you will see that assessing for tenderness is mentioned throughout the book, being a part of the examination of almost every body part and body system, from tapping on a patient's face to test for sinusitis, to pushing on joints to detect arthritis, to pushing on the belly, to pinching the skin to see if the nerves are working properly; and it is used on patients of all ages, from babies to seniors; and on patients who are fully awake to those who are deep in a coma. Why then, is tenderness suddenly invalid when we examine a patient with FM? The answer, I believe, is convenience. Critics of FM find it convenient to disbelieve tenderness in an FM patient, even though they would find it inconvenient to disregard it in a patient complaining of excruciating abdominal pain, because of the medical and medicolegal implications of them missing an acute appendicitis.

Note also that many 'objective' signs of illness can be 'faked'. Fever can be induced by drinking a hot liquid just before coming in to see the doctor. A rapid heart rate and elevated blood pressure can be triggered by rapidly pacing about the room before the doctor walks in; some even can cause it just by working up their own level of anxiety. Rashes, abrasions and swelling can be self-induced, by hitting, scratching, and other self-injurious behaviours. In fact, that more FM patients have not resorted to such behaviours might suggest that faking is not actually on the minds of nearly as many as some critics seem to think.

Finally, with respect to tenderness as a valid sign, in one study, doctors were asked to examine several FM patients and also actors who had been instructed to fake having FM, and the doctors were able to accurately diagnose FM 80% of the time(79). What this means is that there is more than a patient just saying something hurts when pushed on. Clearly, **there are other non-verbal clues during the examination for tenderness that cannot be easily manipulated by someone trying to deceive the doctor.**

So... is tenderness a valid physical sign? Yes. If not, doctors could probably shorten the physical examinations they do by about 20%. And if they eliminated both tenderness and pain brought on with movement (another non-'objective' sign), they could eliminate the lion's share of the musculoskeletal examination. It also would likely put all independent medical examiners out of business.

Fibromyalgia does have objective physical signs

Besides the legitimacy of tenderness as a valid physical finding, believed by the vast majority of doctors in most clinical settings, there have been a handful of physical findings that patients cannot fake or manipulate, identified in those with FM. Most pertain to something called the *autonomic nervous system*, which lends further credence to FM being a disease of the nervous system, and not of the muscles directly.

In Chapter 11, I briefly described the autonomic (involuntary) nervous system. As opposed to nerves that give us sensation and motor control, the autonomic nervous system controls such things as our blood pressure, heart rate, skin temperature, and how much we sweat. As explained earlier, it controls skin temperature by regulating the flow of blood to the skin; and it probably works the same way with sweating.

In several studies comparing FM patients versus healthy individuals, autonomic nervous system irregularities have been evident. These irregularities include:

- *(a)* alterations in skin temperature, being reduced over the back(250), but higher in the hands(251);
- *(b)* orthostatic hypotension, which is inadequate control of blood pressure when someone goes from lying to standing(253) – what normally happens when someone goes from lying to standing is that blood vessels contract to prevent gravity pulling blood away from the brain; in many FM patients, this normal adjustment to changes in body posture is inadequate, so their blood pressure falls excessively and they feel light-headed when they stand; and
- *(c)* *reactive hyperaemia*, which is exaggerated (excessive) blood flow to the skin in response to a briefly-applied painful stimulus (like pinching or a pin prick),

100

causing the skin to go very red once the stimulus is removed, and to stay redder than normal for a prolonged period of time(254;255).

A further, more-recently described objective finding that is apparent in FM patients is called a *nociceptive flexion reflex*. *Nociception* is defined as the nerve processes that underlie the processing and encoding of noxious stimuli, like pain, extreme heat, extreme cold, etc. Using this reflex to study central and chronic pain states has been scientifically validated; it also is useful in determining the effectiveness of various analgesic (pain-killing) drugs(306;307). Using a test called an *electromyelogram* that measures electrical activity in muscle, the reflex is measured as the extent to which a specific muscle in the leg withdraws in response to an electrical stimulus applied directly to the sural nerve of the leg(308). The nociceptive flexion reflex threshold refers to the level of stimulus that generates a measurable withdrawal response. In two studies performed by different research groups, FM patients exhibited a statistically significant decrease in their nociceptive flexion reflex threshold relative to control subjects(309;310); in other words, even at the level of individual nerves and muscle cells, FM patients flinched early to a subtle electrical stimulus.

And a Danish group of researchers has recently published several papers identifying the presence of myofascial trigger points in FM that **(1)** can be felt as taut bands of muscle, like the *Muskelharten* (muscle hardness)(96;97) or *Muskelschwiele* (muscle calluses)(311) described more than 150 years ago in Germany; **(2)** exhibit a local *twitch response* when poked with a needle; (3) demonstrate spontaneous, abnormal electrical activity on electromyelogram (EMG); and (4) appear abnormal when imaged by two-dimensional ultrasound(261-263). If any of these findings can be reproduced by other research groups, it is another reason to maintain the 1990 ACR criteria(81), using tender points as one of the two main criteria used to classify (and diagnose) FM, instead of adopting the most-recently proposed ACR preliminary diagnostic criteria that have dropped all physical findings for diagnosis(83).

In fact, Granges and Littlejohn, in Australia, suggested that four physical findings might be used, in combination, to diagnose FM, the latter two being quite 'objective', with the four criteria together distinguishing those with FM from healthy subjects with 86% accuracy(255). These four findings were: **(1)** *pain threshold to pressure*; **(2)** *skin-fold tenderness* (pinching the skin alone, while not pushing on or pinching underlying muscle or other tissue); **(3)** *reactive skin hyperaemia* (as described above, excessively prolonged skin redness after the examiner pinches the skin); and **(4)** *tissue compliance*, measured with a special calliper (measuring device) over the trapezius muscle of the shoulder (the prominent muscle that stretches from the neck to the shoulder), and in the mid and low back. Granges and Littlejohn concluded that:

"... there are clinical signs, apart from the tender points, which are abnormal in FS that appear to be useful as objective signs in the assessment of patients with FS, whether for diagnostic, therapeutic or research purposes."

Clearly, then, FM patients don't 'look normal' if you look for the right things.

The critic may then say... "Okay, but these are pretty subtle signs. Where's the rash? Where's the fever? Where's the obvious joint swelling?"

To this, I say three letters: P.M.R.

PMR refers to the condition called *polymyalgia rheumatica* that I mentioned in an earlier chapter. PMR is a condition associated with diffuse body pain and stiffness in the absence of all physical signs of illness. A small minority have fever. There also is one blood test that is abnormal, called the *sedimentation rate*, but this is about the least specific lab test available; almost anything makes it go up. AND, even so, the sedimentation rate is normal in about 20% of patients with PMR. Consequently, in

PMR, you have a bunch of usually middle-aged to elderly patients complaining of diffuse pain and stiffness, often in the absence of any objective signs of illness. It can be extremely disabling.

As an example, let me tell you about the first patient I ever saw with PMR. This was at the Veterans Administration Hospital in San Francisco, where I did some of my Internal Medicine training. At age 65, this gentleman had been extremely active; a regular mountain climber, he and his wife actually had plans to attempt, not Mt. Everest, but one of the neighbouring 'smaller' mountains when he retired. But, about 6 months before he retired, he woke up with a stiff shoulder. He thought it had gotten stiff playing tennis. But the next day it was worse. Within a week or so, both shoulders were affected. Within a month, he had stiffness in his low back and hips too, such that he retired from work several months earlier than he'd planned. Within a month of that, he was in a wheelchair, was morbidly depressed, and was losing tremendous amounts of weight. His doctor ran test after test, and then sent him to one specialist after another. By now, everyone was looking for the cancer they hadn't found yet. He and his family were sure that he was dying. I examined him on a Friday afternoon, and presented the case to the supervising arthritis specialist (Rheumatologist). She diagnosed PMR, prescribed a low dose of prednisone, and told him to "Take heart. This will probably help".

On Monday morning, I kid you not, that same patient waltzed into the waiting room carrying a bouquet of flowers and box of chocolates for the doctor. She'd been right. He did, in fact, have PMR; a disorder that is clinically very much like FM, except for one thing... it gets better. In most patients, a low dose of prednisone makes the symptoms all disappear.

What also is critical to know about PMR is that, untreated, a small, but sizeable percentage of patients are at risk for sudden irreversible blindness. So you DON'T want to miss it.

And yet, again, there are NO OBJECTIVE PHYSICAL SIGNS of illness at all in the vast majority of patients. Why don't FM critics have a problem with PMR? The answer, I think, is easy. PMR gets better with treatment that costs pennies a day. If PMR did not respond to treatment and patients stayed disabled (some actually do continue to have symptoms, though usually are improved with prednisone); OR if the treatment for PMR cost $3,000 instead of $5 a month, I think we'd be reading about how controversial PMR is. It all comes down to dollars and a lack of sense.

The concept of fibromyalgia 'control points' makes no sense

Doctors who rule out FM based upon the presence of tenderness at control points seem to imply that these individuals just complain of tenderness everywhere and, hence, must be faking everything... or, at the very least, are exaggerating. In other words, critics are likening FM to a tiger and saying that it isn't real because it's black everywhere.

However, at least five different, published scientific studies have debunked the concept of fibromyalgia control points by demonstrating that FM patients, indeed, are more tender everywhere than those without FM, not just at the 18 ACR criteria points(78-82). In other words, FM is not a tiger. Patients with FM often hurt and are tender virtually everywhere. This is the nature of the disease. As was already explained in the previous chapter, FM appears to be a disease not of the muscles themselves, but of the central nervous system, in particular that part of the nervous system that processes and regulates pain. This derangement of the way in which the body processes potentially painful stimuli often results in magnification of pain anywhere and everywhere in the body.

The 18 tender points used to diagnose FM, in combination with the complaint of widespread body pain, merely help to distinguish patients with FM from individuals with other conditions, such as RA. In other words, FM is more like a black panther, and RA is a tiger. The two species share areas that are black. But the patient with FM also will be black in areas where the RA patient is orange. In other words, if you find that a given patient is very tender over the back of their hands, this may represent FM or RA. Similarly, patients with both diseases may have tender elbows and shoulders. But the FM patient, unlike most RA patients, also will be tender in the tendons just past the elbow. The FM patient, unlike most RA patients, will be tender in the trapezius muscle that runs between the neck and the shoulder. Many FM patients are tender everywhere, just like the panther is black everywhere. To argue that a panther doesn't exist because it is black in areas that a tiger is orange is ludicrous. But this essentially is the argument some examiners, authors, and insurance lawyers sometimes use.

As prominent FM researcher Dr. Fred Wolfe(82) writes: *"Positive control points are a common feature (63%) in FM, and appear to be a marker for a generally low pain threshold rather than a disproportionate increase in severe symptoms or distress. Control point positivity should not be used to disqualify a diagnosis of FM. Control point measurements do not add much to FM diagnosis or assessment and, perhaps, should be abandoned."*

To Sum Up...

In this chapter I have diffused the anti-FM critique that FM doesn't exist because the only finding such individuals have is tenderness, which is a non-objective sign that can be faked. The counter-arguments -- that tenderness is a widely accepted indicator of underlying disease in countless other settings; that there are other objective physical findings in many patients with FM; and that using *control points* to defrock FM makes as much sense as denying the existence of panthers -- all are widely supported by scientific evidence.

To this, zealous critics might say – "So what! None of these physical findings or laboratory abnormalities are SPECIFIC (in other words, exclusive) to fibromyalgia!"

The next two chapters will refute this latest argument.

CHAPTER 12: REASON #9
THE LACK OF SPECIFIC FINDINGS IS <u>NOT</u> UNIQUE TO FIBROMYALGIA

In the field of medical research, the words *specific* and *specificity* have very strict definitions. And to understand what they mean, it also is helpful to know what medical researchers and health care professionals mean when they use the words *sensitive* and *sensitivity* when referring to a particular test or finding.

Sensitivity refers to the percentage of people in a population of interest who a given test or physical finding identifies as diseased. A test is deemed *sensitive* when a high percentage (for example, more than 90%) of people who have the disease have a positive test. In other words, only a small percentage of people with the disease test negative. For example, a particular test called the anti-nuclear antibody (ANA) test is seen in virtually everyone who has a disease called systemic lupus erythematosus (SLE; also just called *lupus*). The sensitivity of the ANA test is more than 99%.

Specificity is very different. Specificity is the percentage of truly non-diseased people who are identified as such by the test or sign. In other words, if you test 100 people who you know DON'T have the disease, and only 1% of them test positive, then the specificity of that test is 99% (100% minus 1%). In medicine, there are many tests and physical signs that are highly sensitive; but highly *specific* tests and signs are much less common.

A good example that is easy to understand is fever. Virtually everyone with meningitis has a fever. But only a very small percentage of people who have a fever have meningitis. Most fevers are associated with a viral flu of some kind; and there are dozens and dozens of other reasons for someone's temperature to go up besides meningitis. So a fever is very sensitive for meningitis, but very, very non-specific. In fact, fever is not very specific for anything, because so many different conditions can cause your body temperature to rise.

This explanation aside, most critics of fibromyalgia use the word *specific* to mean *exclusive*. In other words, they say: "Sure, people with fibromyalgia have all these tender points, but these areas are tender on a lot of people who don't have any pain at all." In other words, some people just don't like being pushed on. Or they say: "Okay. Research shows that serotonin levels are low in patients with FM; but they also are low in people with other things too. Low serotonin isn't SPECIFIC for fibromyalgia."

At face value, this argument seems like it might make sense. But let's look at some other examples of well-accepted diseases with NO SPECIFIC FINDINGS. I've already mentioned PMR in the last chapter. As I stated earlier, the only routine test that ever is abnormal in PMR is the sedimentation rate, which is probably the least specific test medical laboratories do. The list of conditions that can raise your sedimentation rate would go on forever, and would include virtually every type of infection, whether caused by a bacteria, virus, parasite, or fungus; any and all types of cancer; any inflammatory disease; any condition that raises the number of blood cells or amount of protein in your blood; almost any kind of liver disease; and more.

Let's also look at another condition I mentioned at the very start of this chapter: lupus. *Lupus* (formally called *systemic lupus erythematosus*, SLE) is a serious and universally-accepted disease that is characterized, like FM, on the basis of criteria. In SLE, there are eleven criteria, and a patient is said to have *definite lupus* if they have four of them; *probable lupus* if they have three; and *possible lupus* if they have two of the 11 criteria(312). But what are the criteria? For this, just see below, where I have simplified them for those with no or only limited medical backgrounds:

1. Malar rash: This is a characteristic rash on the face that crosses the bridge of the nose into both cheeks to form a shape like a butterfly (hence, it often is

called a *butterfly rash*). It most closely resembles sunburn; and something that is almost indistinguishable from it is a rash called *acne rosacea*. The website WrongDiagnosis(313) lists eleven causes of a malar rash; in other words, ten others besides lupus, and several of them (like acne rosacea) are much more common than lupus. In other words, most people with a rash like this do NOT have lupus. Since many patients with lupus do not have the rash, this sign is neither sensitive nor specific for SLE.

2. Discoid rash: This is a very non-specific rash, the term *discoid* meaning *coin-shaped*. You can see identical rashes with many other conditions, including several different fungal infections. It is most characteristic of something called *discoid lupus* (DLE), a condition that is quite clinically distinct from SLE, and may not represent the same disorder.

3. Photosensitivity: This is an allergy to the sun causing a rash. And this also is not at all exclusive to SLE, as numerous drugs can cause it.

4. Oral ulcers: sores in the mouth. How non-specific is this? The answer is: so low that no one has even bothered to try to estimate it.

5. Arthritis: swollen joints. Up to 15% of the adult population has arthritis somewhere; and a similar pattern of swollen inflamed joints is seen in many different conditions, including rheumatoid arthritis (RA) that is considerably more common than lupus. The overall specificity of inflammatory arthritis for SLE has been estimated at 37%(314).

6. Serositis: This is inflammation of the lining of either the lungs (pleuritis) or heart (pericarditis). Viral pleuritis is not uncommon. And there are many causes of both conditions (pleuritis and pericarditis) besides lupus.

7.   Protein or sediment called *casts* in the urine: Protein can sometimes be detected in the urine of normal, healthy people after vigorous exercise. Admittedly, for lupus, you need to have a fair amount and it must persist; but both proteinuria (protein in urine) and urine casts are seen in dozens of other conditions.

8.   Seizures or psychosis, both of which rarely are indications of lupus.

9.   Some blood derangement: anaemia; low white blood cell count; or low platelet count (platelets are small cells that help the blood clot); all these conditions are seen in many other settings, and none has distinguishing characteristics in lupus.

10.   Abnormal antibodies to one of three things (double-stranded DNA, Sm proteins, or phospholipid): These are, perhaps, the most *specific* findings in lupus, with *anti-double-stranded DNA antibodies* the best of the three. However, in one study performed on 441 persons with anti-double-stranded DNA antibodies followed for several years, only 85% ever developed lupus(315), meaning that the specificity of this test was only 85%, minimally better than the 81% for the ACR fibromyalgia criteria. Anti-Sm antibodies can be induced by exposure to the Ebstein-Barr virus(316), which is widespread. Anti-phospholipid antibodies are primarily seen in a disorder called *anti-phospholipid antibody (APLA) syndrome*, rather than lupus. And none of these three tests is positive in any more than a minority of SLE patients; so they all are less sensitive for lupus than flipping a coin.

11.   A positive *anti-nuclear anti-body (ANA) test:* Let's especially look at the ANA test, which is positive in anywhere from 5 to 10% of normal, healthy people, or 50 to 100 people out of every thousand. Considering that lupus only affects about one in 1,000, that means that, if you have 1,000 people and test them

for ANA, on average, 50 to 100 of them will have a positive ANA, but only one of those 50 to 100 who have a positive ANA actually will have lupus, which translates into a positive predictive value (which is specificity when tested in the general population) of between one and two percent. In rheumatology clinics, among patients with inflammatory arthritis (who look like they MIGHT have lupus), though 99% sensitive, the specificity of the ANA test has been estimated at less than 50%(314); this, again, is less reliable than flipping a coin.

Technically, then, a person could be diagnosed with *probable lupus* if they are psychotic, have a sun allergy, and have a positive result on a test that, when positive, is less often right than flipping a coin when examined among patients seen in an arthritis clinic. Throw in one other criteria (to make four positive criteria), and that person has *definite lupus*. Overall, the ACR criteria for lupus have a specificity of about 89%(317;318), meaning they wrongly diagnose SLE more than 10% of the time, which could hardly be considered exclusive. In truth, however, this is not nearly as bad as it sounds, because patients who look enough like lupus to meet the criteria but don't have it probably have something close enough that treatment will be much the same, at least initially. Nonetheless, there have been calls to throw away the current SLE criteria because of numerous problems with them(317;318). In other words, it isn't just the FM criteria that have limitations and detractors.

The sad fact is that few medical tests or findings are exclusive to any one disorder, or even highly specific. Diagnoses usually are made on the basis of the doctor or doctors looking at ALL THE EVIDENCE before them, and deciding what is most likely. For many disorders, confirmation comes either from a response to treatment (as with PMR), or from the disease just going away on its own (like the typical viral flu).

If critics insist that any lack of exclusive (or at least highly specific) tests or findings is justification for discarding certain diagnostic labels, then we'd probably have to weed out over 50% of the contents of all our medical text books.

111

A few final words: about labels

I will be discussing the issue of labelling in a later chapter, but some understanding is appropriate here. As I've stated before in Chapter 8, there is a myth in medicine that we have 999 diseases; but the truth is that we have 999 disease labels. Some of these labels, such as pneumococcal pneumonia or gout, work very well. FM, SLE, RA, PMR, and many other disorders that fall under the rheumatic disease umbrella are not well labelled. Lupus has been called the disease of a thousand faces(319) because every patient looks so different. Is lupus all one disease? Or is it actually three diseases; or five; or 100? In fact, we don't know. For now, we must rely on criteria that were created for the disorder by doctors with tremendous experience and insight dealing with this subset of patients; and on common sense. **The exact same thing is true of FM.**

The ACR criteria for FM are about 89% sensitive and 81% specific, making them almost as good as the criteria for rheumatic disorders like rheumatoid arthritis(201). The numerous abnormalities identified in FM patients through research paint a rapidly clarifying picture of a central nervous system disorder that affects different areas of the brain and different chemicals in the brain and nerves that are responsible for sleep, pain perception, and some cognitive functions. This is a much better explanation than we have for disorders like PMR or, as another example, autism(320). And I challenge ANY fibromyalgia critic to go up to the parents of a diagnosed autistic child and tell them that their child is just faking everything.

CHAPTER 13: REASON #10
THERE HAVE BEEN MANY SIMILAR EXAMPLES
IN HISTORY

I've already described numerous disorders that are similar to FM, in terms of having criteria that were developed using the same research methodology as for the FM criteria (e.g., rheumatoid arthritis, lupus); having no hard physical findings (e.g., polymyalgia rheumatica, autism); using tenderness as a major diagnostic clue (e.g., appendicitis, rheumatoid arthritis, and countless others); or having signs and/or test results that are no to little more exclusive than the legions of research-detected abnormalities that have been identified in FM (e.g., lupus, PMR, RA). What I want to do here is look back at history, to see what it shows us about mistakes that have been made in the past by naysayers similar to those currently criticizing FM.

One good example is multiple sclerosis. At one time called *creeping paralysis*, it was first described in the 13th or 14th century. However, it was not recognized as a disease until 1868. For centuries, it was ascribed to hysteria, especially because it was more common in women and most doctors were men(321). Despite evidence of peculiar spinal cord damage in the spine of a patient who died in 1838 of what we now call MS, discovered by Drs. Robert Carswell and Jean Cruveilhier, and subsequent research identifying inflammation of the spinal cord [in 1868], abnormalities in spinal fluid [in 1906], development of an experimental rat model of MS [in 1933], and formation of the United States National Multiple Sclerosis Society [in 1946], it was not until over 100 years after Carswell and Cruveilhier's report that a symposium was held, in 1950 in New York City, at which time a consensus was reached that MS is truly a physical and not just a mental disease(321). Even with this, there remained a subset of patients who had what is called *relapsing-remitting MS* (symptoms and signs would come and then would disappear days or weeks later, in a repeating pattern), who still were felt to be malingerers and/or hysterical until the development of modern advanced imaging techniques (like the MRI) in the 1980s. And it was only in 2007 that the European MS Platform, backed by European parliament, officially demanded equal rights for MS patients.

Crohn's disease and rheumatoid arthritis are among many other examples of now universally-accepted diseases that, as recently as the 1950s, were believed to be either psychogenic or significantly influenced by one's psychological state. And, though now it is common practice to screen for and treat a bacterium called *Helicobacter pylori* for peptic ulcer disease, it was less than 20 years ago that Dr. Barry Marshall, an Australian doctor who suggested that at least some stomach ulcers could be treated with antibiotics, was almost unanimously called a quack.

What can and should we learn from this?

In answer, I refer back to something that was told to me back in 1981, during the first medical school lecture that I ever attended. The speaker said this:

"Fifty percent of what you learn over the next four years will be proven wrong in the next twenty. The problem is: no one can say which 50% will be wrong."

There are numerous other examples of conditions, like multiple sclerosis, that were not believed or felt to be purely psychological disorders until medical technology developed either the diagnostic tools to diagnose them with greater certainty, or highly effective treatments that, through their effectiveness, also validated the disorder's existence.

How were people with underactive thyroid glands treated, if they had no gland enlargement, in the days prior to our being able to measure thyroid hormone levels in blood? Most of these patients were women. Because thyroid hormone regulates the speed of our body's metabolism, such patients complained of a profound lack of energy, and most gained considerable weight. Many were depressed. What do you want to bet

114

that many, if not almost all of these women, were told they just were depressed (or lazy)? All they needed to do was exercise, lose weight, and stop being so depressed (or lazy).

Does this sound familiar? From my past experience treating hundreds and hundreds of FM patients over several years, I suspect that most FM patients have been told these same things, if not by their own doctor, then by some doctor they were referred to, perhaps for a disability or work assessment.

My question is: why do we have to keep making the same mistake?

Or, as Bob Dylan wrote,

How many times can a man turn his head
and pretend that he just doesn't see?

Blowin' in the Wind

CHAPTER 14: REASON #11
IT'S NOT AN ISSUE OF LABELLING

There are critics who believe that patients with FM only are sick because someone has told them that they are; that, by giving someone a label for their symptoms, we perpetuate those symptoms and make the patient worse. One such critic wrote:

"When one has tuberculosis, one has tuberculosis, whether or not it is diagnosed. The same is true for cancer, rheumatoid arthritis, hookworm infestation—really, of the gamut of diseases. But not for fibromyalgia (FM). No one has FM until it is diagnosed."(111)

This statement can be interpreted in several different ways. It implies:

1. that tuberculosis, rheumatoid arthritis, hookworm, and every other disease has a level of objectivity that FM lacks;

2. that the patients given the FM label are just those who are at the upper end of the normal aches and pains and fatigue that everyone has;

3. that those given the label of FM are just those who can't cope with these normal aches and pains, and who then complain long and loud enough to be labelled; and

4. that giving someone the label of *fibromyalgia* actually makes them sick.

Let's look at the first three arguments only briefly, because the first two have been debunked earlier in this book, and the third will be covered extensively in the next chapter.

All other diseases have a level of objectivity that FM lacks

The contention that all other diseases except FM have irrefutable, objective evidence to support their existence even before diagnosis in each and every patient is nonsense. Countering the above-mentioned 'real disease' examples, starting with tuberculosis, note that tuberculosis is an organism, not a disease. There are many, many individuals who are tuberculosis carriers who have no knowledge of their illness, have no symptoms, and receive no treatment. Are these patients sick? Do they have 'tuberculosis'? If so, should we not be forced to identify every potentially-pathogenic bacteria or other organism in every living being on the planet, and label each individual who has any potentially disease-causing organism ill? If we did this, we ALL would have personal medical history lists pages and pages long, because there isn't a person on the planet who EVER has been totally free of all potentially pathogenic organisms.

And, as already discussed, rheumatoid arthritis is a diagnosis that typically is made using criteria not unlike those used by most doctors to diagnose FM(201). When assessing a patient with possible RA, examiners utilize a checklist of seven items to estimate the patient's probability of disease. There is no gold standard test that absolutely confirms rheumatoid arthritis. Although some mistakenly attribute the presence of an antibody called *rheumatoid factor* in a patient's serum to be confirmatory, in fact it is far from being such, since 5% of healthy adults, according to the way in which the rheumatoid factor test is defined, have an elevated level of rheumatoid factor in their blood? Of these, at most 20% ever will ultimately develop joint symptoms consistent with RA(322). Every practicing rheumatologist has seen numerous patients who complain of significant joint pain and stiffness, without any clear, objective joint swelling or other findings, on physical examination, blood test or radiograph. Do these patients have rheumatoid arthritis? Some may receive the diagnosis, only to have all symptoms resolve spontaneously over weeks, months or years, without requiring further treatment. Did they ever have RA? Others may be felt not to have adequate evidence of RA initially to justify a diagnosis, only to have it clearly express itself later.

Clearly then, saying that FM does not exist until it is diagnosed while every other condition exists as soon as symptoms start, is misguided at best.

The FM label is only given to those with the upper range of normal aches and pains

This second perspective implies that patients diagnosed with FM are just those either at the top end of the normal spectrum, or who just cannot cope. They may have more aches and pain, but are otherwise no different than those who have fewer aches and pains. That aches and pains and fatigue and difficulty sleeping are common, almost ubiquitous, problems in society is used as an argument to invalidate any individuals who report more of them than usual. Again, these people just can't cope.

In our own survey of 3,400 non-institutionalized adults in London, Ontario, 36% of females and 33% of males reported having some pain in muscles, bones or joints that had lasted at least one week over the preceding three months(13;323). Sixty percent of females and 45 percent of males reported having had frequent fatigue. In other surveys, men have tenderness at an average of between 3 and 4 of the so-called fibromyalgia tender points, and women at between 5 and 6 of these points. So what makes FM so different from what the general population of healthy adults has? The answer is: not just the severity and distribution of their pain and tenderness, but also the severity and number of other symptoms.

First of all, just because some value lies on a continuum does not make it normal. There is a broad distribution of blood pressures, but we still treat individuals who have blood pressures of 160 over 100; in fact, doctors generally consider treating any systolic blood pressure above 140 and most diastolic values over 90. The same broad range exists for blood sugars; yet no one denies that diabetes exists.

Technically, any individual who has pain in his or her right shoulder, extending into the shoulder blade, and soreness of the left toe, meets the first 1990 American College of Rheumatology (ACR) criterion for FM(81), which calls for 'widespread' pain. This person has pain above and below the waist, on the right and left side, and affecting both the trunk and the limbs. However, there are several features that distinguish this individual from the person with FM, and virtually no astute clinician would ever even consider FM in this patient.

As stated in Chapter 1 and elsewhere in this book, the person with FM complains of generalized pain, often aching all over. They also report severe, debilitating fatigue, non-restorative sleep, and other symptoms. They are diffusely tender. Individuals with this constellation of symptoms plus the generalized tenderness are clinically distinct from the person with pain here and there who is somewhat tired sometimes. This is obvious clinically, and it has been proven in various studies of the general population(197-199). It also has been demonstrated by an almost endless string of research studies that have detected other abnormalities in those with the FM label, as discussed in detail in Chapters 10 through 12.

The FM label is only given to those who can't cope with the normal aches and fatigue everyone else lives with

This argument will be countered extensively in the next chapter, so I will speak no further of it here.

Labelling someone with FM actually makes them sick

This is the main argument I want to defrock in this chapter. But first, let me explain what actually is being implied in greater detail. For a variety of reasons, the labelling of certain chronic pain patients as having FM has sparked concern that the label of fibromyalgia, in itself, might precipitate or exacerbate behaviour that has been variably termed *illness behaviour, learned pain*(324) and *learned helplessness*(325). In other words, if you tell people they are sick, they will act sick, even if they truly are not. This potentially results in increased symptoms, worsened function, increased disability claims, and increased health care-seeking behaviour(27;91;326). A case for the danger of labelling has been made for *black lung disease* as it occurred in coal mining areas in the United States. In this example, large numbers of miners were labelled with black lung disease and granted disability pensions based on X-ray findings, despite entirely normal lung function when tested for it (7).

To date, however, there is no good evidence that the FM label has either a deleterious or beneficial effect. In fact, the only study that has been done to examine this claim generated results that argue against the label itself negatively influencing outcomes. In this study, which we did in London, Ontario, we first compared 72 persons with FM who had been previously-undiagnosed, against 28 previously diagnosed FM cases, all identified within a general population survey(92); in other words, these people were randomly identified in the community through a scientifically-validated general population screening procedure(327). We then followed the 72 newly-diagnosed individuals for three years, re-assessing them at 18 months and 36 months to see how they compared at those times versus how they were the day we first met and diagnosed them. If the label of fibromyalgia truly makes people worse, then these 72 people should, on average, have been worse at these 18 and 36 month assessments. But they were not. In fact, if anything, over time, newly-diagnosed individuals with FM may have improved slightly, reporting fewer symptoms and being less dissatisfied with their health. Interestingly, at the first visit, the 28 who already had been diagnosed with FM when we first saw them were worse than the 72 not previously diagnosed, suggesting this:

Instead of the FM label making people worse, as some have claimed(27;77;91;326), those who have worse symptoms tend to be diagnosed with FM sooner.

This, in fact, is what one would expect of all legitimate diseases. Shouldn't one expect the person with worse heart disease to come to the doctor first? Or the person whose diabetes develops with a very rapid rise in blood sugars to come to the doctor before someone whose blood sugars only rise very slowly? Or someone with a rapidly-growing, aggressive and spreading cancer to be seen, on average, earlier than someone with a slow-growing tumour? The answer to all these questions is the same: of course.

Strengths of the London study mentioned above are that this was a study of people randomly selected from the general population, and NOT patients already being seen in a specialty clinic, which allowed us to truly see the effect of labelling.

Our findings are in direct contrast to the opinions of those who suggest abolishing the FM label for something 'more neutral'(26;98;328;329). But these contradictory authors fail to offer scientific evidence supporting their claims. One author's 'critical appraisal of the fibromyalgia concept' is anything but, because he doesn't even make an attempt to either perform research in the area or review the research of others. It's like someone saying: "I've thought about it, and thought about it, and decided that the cure to all disease is apple juice." Okay... but based on what?

Some have reported that the FM label has resulted in an epidemic of FM(62;329), but there is no evidence of this. The only study that has looked at the incidence of new cases of FM over time was conducted in Finland, and no increase was noted. What likely is happening to create the impression that FM is more common than it used to be is that there now is increased recognition of FM by health care practitioners. The same phenomenon exists when you buy a new car... suddenly you see more cars of the same make on the road than you ever noticed before. Do you truly believe that more people suddenly decide to buy that very same make of car the very same day you do?

Other authors present detailed, anecdotal accounts of patients who, once labelled, "are drawn into medicalization and dependency"(76) and "become victims worthy of a star appearance on the Oprah Winfrey show"(330). The results of our study do not eliminate the possibility that a minority of patients labelled with fibromyalgia become obsessed with their illness, leading to increased illness behaviour. However, the same might be said of certain patients labelled with high blood pressure, heart disease, or a long list of other conditions.

It may be that, in certain settings, like the person applying for a disability pension or compensation after an injury, the FM label may contribute to heightened illness behaviour and, hence, might be problematic(62); but such an assumption is unproven. We did not specifically address this issue in our study, because it would have required a much larger number of newly-diagnosed, community FM cases and, hence, many more than the already 3,400 interviews that we undertook. Moreover, although the percentage of our FM cases claiming total disability did increase from 23% to 35% after labelling (a difference that was not statistically significant), one must not ignore the following fact:

Two-thirds of our newly-diagnosed FM cases failed to consider themselves totally disabled over a 3-year period.

This suggests that the FM label did not result in a rush of disability claims. Again, our newly-labelled subjects reported fewer symptoms, fewer major symptoms, and less dissatisfaction with health after three years. In other words, making patients worse does not appear to be a significant problem with the FM label.

To say one last thing about the person with FM applying for disability payments, however: how is such a person supposed to behave? Insurance companies increasingly want you to 'prove' that you truly are disabled, and so do courts. If you truly are disabled, why would you possibly try to show that you aren't? Would anyone advise a badly dyslexic person to repeatedly deny their dyslexia when questioned about their poor reading and writing skills? Or the person with angina to hide their chest pain and pretend it doesn't exist?

As I have said for years and throughout this book, for a host of bad reasons, those who have FM are consistently held up to a different standard than persons with almost any other disorder. When is this going to stop?

CHAPTER 15: REASON #12
THE MENTAL-VERSUS-PHYSICAL ARGUMENT
DOESN'T WORK

A final, often-used argument against FM is that it all is just a mental, or psychological, disease:

> Sure, these patients are everywhere. Sure, everyone seems to get it. Sure, everyone seems alike. Sure, these patients have various 'objective' physical and biochemical findings and changes in brain blood flow. And maybe the fibromyalgia label doesn't make them worse.

> But the same might all be said of major depression. That's why we treat depression with medication. And it is undeniable that many FM patients are psychologically distressed, with some suffering from major depression. This relatively high prevalence of depression has led some to conclude that FM is a psychiatric disorder manifested by physical symptoms(331;332). In other words, all FM really is, is a form of depression, or some other psychological distress.

This argument may seem enticing because, again, many, many FM patients are depressed. Admittedly, I think most people would feel depressed or stressed if they felt really sick and no one believed them, and their insurance company refused to pay them, and some doctors actually told them (or treated them like) they were faking. But, this aside, there are several counter-arguments against the 'FM is just psychological' claim. They include:

1. Psychological disease is real too;

2. Not all persons with FM are psychologically distressed; and

3. The mental versus physical dichotomy of disease just doesn't work.

Psychological disease is real too

This is an anti-critic counter-argument that the naysayers sometimes hand us on a platter, when they insist that the various chemical changes seen in FM can be seen in depressed patients too. What this means is that, as most doctors and researchers have known for years, there is a chemical basis behind depression and probably most so-called 'mental illnesses'. And if they are accepted as real, why shouldn't FM be?

In medical school, doctors are taught that, at every second of every day, from the time an embryo is conceived (in fact, even beforehand in the as-yet unfertilized egg and sperm) through to the time of one's death (and for some time afterwards), chemical reactions are occurring... millions and maybe even billions of them... such reactions occurring constantly in every living cell. And that these reactions are behind everything we do or feel or think. As stated repeatedly throughout this book, FM critics seem to argue this as one of their main reasons that FM doesn't exist... that such chemical changes cannot be found and/or confirmed in FM. So... if chemical reactions underlie everything we do, feel, or think, how can we possibly distinguish between physical and psychological disease? Both have underlying chemical changes that are abnormal or, at the very least, dysfunctional.

Think about a wrist watch or clock. These days, almost everything is digital, but specifically think of one of those fine Swiss watches with a minute and hour hand, and maybe even a second hand. If you opened one of these watches and looked closely at all the inner workings, you'd see that the watch contains a complex system of gears and levers, all moving in perfect synchronization.

Saying that one's depression is not physiologically based is akin to saying that your Swiss watch is running slow just because it wants to. Imagine bringing your watch to the jeweller because it's running slow. Could you imagine the jeweller, confirming that the watch is running slow, and then opening it up, looking at it for awhile and finally telling you that "everything is running fine"? You'd say: "Really? Then why is my watch not running right?"

That question, in fact, is what FM researchers are asking... why are people with FM, to continue the watch analogy, not running properly. We know, from the evidence given in the next section, that depression or anxiety **does not** universally **cause** FM. Depression *might* make symptoms worse in some, or even possibly be causative in a minority of patients. But all this is irrelevant; because, irrespective of the role or lack of role of depression or anxiety, just like the Swiss watch that's running slow, the body of the FM patient is not functioning properly. Based upon what doctors-in-training are taught in medical school, this means that there is some underlying chemical and/or physiological abnormality.

I'll say a bit more about all this later, when I discuss something called the *biopsychosocial model.*

Not all persons with FM are psychologically distressed

If, in fact, FM is merely a manifestation of psychological disease or distress – if this is the actual CAUSE – then it follows that EVERYONE with FM should be psychologically distressed. But such is NOT the case. In no study that has been done assessing either psychiatric disorders alone or the full range of FM symptoms, have depression, anxiety, and other evidence of psychological distress been identified in ALL individuals(3;14;15;23;108;136;154;161;189;196;197;199;333-345). Rates in the clinic have varied, but generally all fall below 50%. In our own general population survey, among 100 adults confirmed to have fibromyalgia, less than one in three reported depression as a major problem(197); similarly, fewer than one in three reported significant anxiety(197); and most of the patients who reported one, also reported the other. In other words, a significant minority reported depression AND anxiety, but most of the remainder reported neither.

Our percentages of self-rated significant depression and anxiety are lower than those reported in most other studies, likely for this reason: we studied people with FM outside of a specialty clinic, recruiting them randomly from the general population of London, Ontario by doing almost 3,400 telephone interviews. Consequently, we assessed the full range of fibromyalgia, including those whose symptoms were mild enough, or who were coping well enough, or who were early enough in their disease that they hadn't yet been referred to and/or seen by a specialist. Again, if psychological distress was the underlying CAUSE of FM, every one of our FM subjects should have reported feeling depressed, anxious, or in some other way psychologically disturbed. But they certainly did not report this. It is possible that some were depressed or anxious and did not admit it; but why would more than a few, if any, do this? What possibly could have been the motive for persons with FM, en masse, to do this?

We also didn't just ask these individuals if they were anxious, depressed, or stressed. We used scientifically-validated screening questionnaires for anxiety and depression: specifically the Center for Epidemiological Studies Depression (CES-D) scale(346) and the State-Trait Anxiety Inventory (STAI)(347).

Other researchers have looked at the association between psychiatric symptoms and FM and, when compared with rheumatoid arthritis (RA), another painful disorder that happens to be associated with objective swelling and damage to joints, in five of eleven studies, the rate of depression was no different between the two disorders (333;334;336;337;340). In short, then, the evidence is clear that FM is not universally accompanied by depression, anxiety, or some other psychological disturbance. Rather, at least a significant portion of any psychological distress that exists seems to be related to the chronic pain, disability, and/or other symptoms; and I suspect that a good deal more relates (1) to the lack of acceptance many of these patients feel because others don't seem to believe them; and (2) to the consequences of that lack of acceptance, like living in poverty because their applications for disability payments repeatedly are denied.

Here's a story for you: I once had a patient who had moved to Canada from Poland in his mid twenties to forge a better life for his wife and family. University-trained as an electrical engineer in Poland, his credentials were not accepted in North America, so he eventually got a job working at a factory. Everyone at the factory knew about the hazardous working conditions, largely stemming from the incredibly heavy barrels of oil that had to be moved around, and the shockingly old and weak raised wooden platforms (or *pallets*) upon which they were stored. One day after he'd worked at the factory for six years without taking a single sick day, while he was rolling a barrel into place onto one of these wooden pallets, since it was far too heavy to lift, the barrel broke through, along with the man's foot. The barrel falling towards him, he twisted as far as he could to get out of the way, lest he be crushed and killed. He tore every ligament in his knee and wrenched his back so badly he couldn't even get up without assistance. I met him about two years later. His knee had required two surgeries, but still was obviously swollen; and, though he NEVER complained of his knee, he walked slowly and with an unmistakeable limp. His back caused him so much pain he still had to go to therapy three times a week. And he hurt everywhere else too, this having developed within about 2-3 months of the accident.

After he'd been off of work for six months, his employer told him that he had to show up for work on Monday or be fired. He tried, lasted about half a day, and then had to be helped to a car and driven home. His employer fired him on the spot. At the time I saw him, he still hurt almost everywhere, but especially in his low back. He had 16 of 18 fibromyalgia tender points, was sleeping very poorly, was always exhausted, had daily headaches, and had trouble some days remembering anything. I diagnosed him with post-traumatic fibromyalgia.

To that date, he hadn't received one dime in compensation from the company; they claimed that the accident was his fault, despite prior written complaints from the workers about the thin wooden pallets that the barrels were stored on. And he had repeatedly been denied disability payments from the government. He and his wife had had to sell the home they'd bought just a year before his injury. They no longer had a car, because they couldn't afford one. They now lived with their two children (they were about six and eight years old, if I recall correctly) in a one-bedroom apartment; his wife shared a big bed with the kids; he slept on a mattress on the floor in the living room. The only money they had coming in was from his wife's part time, minimum-wage job, and from him working a few hours a week (because that was all his back would tolerate) helping a friend out by working behind the counter at a small store. For Christmas that year, the children each received a single pack of gum.

And, get this... he wasn't depressed. He smiled throughout his time with me, happy to finally be seen by someone he thought could help him. Yes... he wished his life would get better. He felt sorry that he couldn't provide better for his children. He missed working. He missed the friends he'd made at work. He missed the family he'd left back in Poland. But he wasn't depressed, or anxious, or panicky, or hysterical. He loved his wife and children, and was so grateful they'd stayed with him through all this. He appreciated the one friend who had given him work. He loved living in Canada. He was so appreciative of me that, at his next visit, he brought me a plate of delicious cookies that his wife had baked for me. And he was hopeful that, one day, his life would get better. I remember him saying: "So many are so much worse off than I am."

The strength of this man's character, in my opinion, would put 99% of the rest of us to shame. He had found a way to cope with a mountain of injustices so extreme it would cause most people to absolutely explode.

He is just one example of the many patients I have met who prove to me that FM is not just psychological decompensation in response to stress. And a third counter-argument against FM just being psychological is this:

The mental-versus-physical dichotomy of disease doesn't work

Many doctors do this: they first look for objective evidence of physical disease, by examination, laboratory test, and X-ray or some other imaging technique (like CAT scan or MRI). If they find some, they consider the patient's problem a physical one; but if they don't, then it MUST all be in the patient's head. In other words, the more likely it's physical disease, the less likely that it's mental disease. It's almost like a teeter-totter (some call it a see-saw); as one end goes up, the other end MUST come down.

My question is: When are we finally going to discard the outdated concept that psychological and physical illnesses are opposites?

A huge body of research tells us that psychological and physical ill health move, not in opposite directions, but in tandem. The two are NOT opposite ends of a teeter-totter; they rise and fall together.

What chronic illness does not affect us psychologically? Are newly-diagnosed cancer patients not psychologically distraught? What about recent stroke victims? In fact, the stress levels of new stroke victims in a rehabilitation unit have been shown to be very high(348). Is this surprising? How many coherent patients do you think could be told they have cancer, or could wake up in the hospital unable to speak or move their right arm and leg, without feeling some level of anxiety, depression, or both? Does this make cancer and stroke psychological diseases? They're both just in the patient's head? Of course not! To even think this is absurd.

Rheumatoid arthritis patients also have high levels of psychological distress, with major depression affecting up to one in three patients(333). Is this surprising? Many RA patients have widespread pain and significant functional limitations because of it. Given that many of these patients were quite healthy prior to the onset of their RA, and given that many still are relatively young, it is totally understandable that many would feel depressed, or anxious or both. And all these things can be said of FM, as well.

131

The reality is that severe physical illness often causes severe emotional stress. And, in the same way, chronic physical illness begets chronic psychological distress, and *vice versa*. Numerous research studies have demonstrated alterations in body functions at a chemical (physiological) level, including decreased function of the immune system, among those who are depressed(349-352). The dramatic increase in death rates in the year following the death of a spouse(353-355) is further, poignant evidence that psychological distress affects us physically.

Moreover, as stated earlier, so-called 'psychological disorders' are not without chemical and other microscopic changes that occur in the brain and elsewhere. Such changes have been identified in numerous psychiatric diagnoses including schizophrenia, major depression, bipolar disorder, obsessive-compulsive disorder, and attention deficit hyperactivity disorder, to name a few; and many of these changes have been behind the various drug therapies that have been developed.

As such, the distinction between physical and psychological illness becomes increasingly meaningless. The distinction between a physical symptom and a psychological one becomes more blurred. What is important is that all such patients are in distress, and that physicians can choose either to help or, I am saddened to say, hinder them.

This association between mind and body health is all part of what has been termed the *biopsychosocial model* of illness, a concept that is far better supported by current research than the biomedical model so many doctors were taught in medical school. In short, the *biomedical model* sees disease as a combination of biochemical or anatomical changes in the body and the resultant tissue damage that stems from them. On the other hand:

The biopsychosocial model sees all disease as interactions between what is happening inside a person's body (chemically and anatomically; the *bio* component of biopsychosocial); how that person feels, both physically and emotionally (the *psycho* component); and how all of this affects how they function, at home and in society (the *social* component.

One of my sons broke his wrist playing competitive hockey in the second last game of the season two years, and had to have it placed in a cast. His six weeks in a cast was certainly inconvenient for him, to be sure. But he also had the fun of having all his teammates and friends, including all the girls at school, sign it. In short, he became a bit of a celebrity. He also got out of some homework and a few house chores because of it. And he quickly figured out which video games he could play well with one hand. All in all, I think he coped pretty well. But if my brother Donald, who is a concert pianist, broke his wrist, I expect that the experience would be entirely different. The same injury, but different social conditions, would drastically influence how that injury would be experienced.

Again, to most people, I would think that all of this makes sense. But, somehow, it does not appear to, to many FM critics, who see disease as either physical OR mental.

The biopsychosocial model was not designed to apply just to chronic pain conditions. It probably applies to all illness. Even in the setting of a short-lived, entirely reversible physical illness, there likely is some increase in the risk of emotional distress. How many of us get upset and irritable when we have a bad cold? But the risk of psychological disturbance intuitively should be greater for chronic conditions that either worsen or don't get better. An additional contributing factor may be the health care system itself. Those who have chronic, non-remitting disorders likely will be exposed to more health care services over a greater period of time than patients with acute disease that resolves quickly. Such health-care system induced stress may be particularly common in conditions like FM, because such patients often perceive hostility or indifference in some health care providers, or feel that the explanations they receive for their symptoms are inadequate.

SUMMARY

Over the last 12 chapters, I have provided at least 12 solid and scientifically-supported reasons why fibromyalgia is real and/or why it is being held up to a grossly unfair level of scrutiny. Whether the label *fibromyalgia* is a good one; whether the way we currently diagnose it stands up to the test of time; whether FM represents one disease or a spectrum of disease – all of this is irrelevant. What is relevant is that the arguments that those who suffer from FM have legitimate, physiologically-based disease far, far, far overshadow all arguments to the contrary.

To this, critics then might say: "But what about common sense?" If you read the numerous editorials that have been written by anti-FM critics, one relatively consistent approach these authors use is to implore the reader and the entire medical community to "just use common sense. Let's be reasonable about this." By this, they seem to say: "if you don't see anything, c'mon... it just isn't there!"

BUT, what really doesn't make sense, and what truly is NOT reasonable is to walk through life constantly wearing a blindfold, while insisting that it's everyone else who can't see.

And this brings me back to the question of why? Why are certain physicians so zealous in their anti-FM sentiments that they insist upon blindly and repeatedly thrusting their opinions upon the general and medical community, through both the spoken and written word? I cannot speak for all of them. But I will quote one of my colleagues who commented: "It probably pays a lot better to be an FM critic than to be an FM supporter." Those who do FM research receive no extra salary for their findings if they turn out one way or the other; and researchers are obligated to report negative findings. Fabricating findings to support one's pre-determined conclusions, and this being discovered, may ruin one's career in research. You'd never be awarded a research grant ever again.

Moreover, research grants are becoming increasing difficult to get, and the preparation of grant applications takes huge amounts of time (weeks or months per grant), with no guarantees of success. And, even if successful at winning a research grant, very rarely does the researcher himself or herself receive any personal pay from the grant; and successful grant applicants frequently are awarded less money than they originally asked for, meaning that they have to do more with less, and sometimes end up supplementing the grant from their own personal income. I can truthfully say that my research lost me income, primarily because it removed me from the clinic where I made money on a fee-for-service basis. And, on occasion, I was looked upon with disdain: why didn't I study some 'legitimate disease' like lupus or rheumatoid arthritis?

Meanwhile, those who merely postulate with a pen lose far less time from their money-making ventures than those conducting scientific research. Their papers are easy to write, because they require little to no review of the published medical literature (I once read an anti-FM editorial that contained a grand total of three references, all of which were earlier opinion papers written by the same author who was writing the editorial). And many of these papers are rehashes of earlier published versions written by the same author – reworded and re-organized, but quoting many of the same non-scientific references and making the same general points.

Hence, if I were to come up with a thirteenth reason why FM is real, it would be this:

FM is real because no FM researcher benefits personally from saying so, other than from feeling the personal satisfaction of unveiling the truth and helping a forgotten number of patients who truly need and deserve help.

PART 3

TRAUMA,

DISABILITY,

AND

DYLAN

CHAPTER 16

TRAUMA AND FIBROMYALGIA: IS THERE AN ASSOCIATION AND WHAT DOES IT MEAN?

For more than two decades, some have suspected that at least some cases of fibromyalgia (FM) are associated with a recent injury(356). More recently, several authors have argued that an injury actually might CAUSE FM. These authors, who include Bennett(357), Greenfield(18), Romano(358) and Waylonis(359), all have characterized what has since been called *post-traumatic* or *reactive* FM (as in, some reaction to an injury). Bennett has claimed that FM symptoms, if they are to occur, can develop up to 18 months after an injury has taken place(357). Greenfield and Waylonis have noted that those who have FM that started following an injury ultimately do worse(18;359). Between 25% and 50% of people with FM recall some event that immediately preceded the onset of their symptoms; and, most often, that event was some form of physical injury(18;197). On the other hand, many are highly critical of the concept of post-traumatic FM(26;360).

The primary objective of this chapter, then, is to review the research that has been done, so as to answer the following two questions:

1. Is there an association between past injury and FM?
2. If so, what does it mean?

Why is an association between injury and FM important?

There are several reasons why a chapter reviewing the association between trauma and FM is important in a book such as this. First, FM has a huge impact both upon the individual who has it and upon society. Second, there are numerous critical implications of a trauma-FM association; for example, related to the issues of preventing it, treating it early, performing other research into what causes FM, and resolving disability and compensation cases. Third and finally, there actually is evidence that such an association might exist. Let's explore these three reasons in greater detail.

1. FM has a large impact upon both the individual and society

As stated earlier in this book, FM has emerged as a significant worldwide health problem. As reviewed extensively in Chapters 5 and 6, it appears to be everywhere and to affect all ages, races, and backgrounds. Not only that, but it is one of the most common conditions seen in outpatient arthritis (rheumatology) clinics around the world. This includes Canada(361), the United States(362), Mexico(129), Spain(363), Australia(364), and elsewhere. It also accounts for about one in 40 patients seen in family practice clinics(365), and about one in 18 seen in general medicine clinics(14). If the figures identified in London Ontario and Arendal Norway represent what happens elsewhere, on average, up to one in ten women will develop FM in her lifetime(13;128), with roughly one in 200 women coming down with FM each year(366). It also appears not to be at all uncommon in children(151;178) (please refer back to Chapter 6 for more on FM in children).

Fibromyalgia can impact the individual who has it in many ways, worsening both their quality of life and their function. Patients with FM report disabilities in their daily activities that are as extensive as those reported by patients with rheumatoid arthritis (RA), and more extensive than those reported by patients with osteoarthritis (OA), the most common form of arthritis(367). They rate their quality of life as lower than patients with either RA or OA(368). They report lower overall health and function and greater pain than patients with RA, OA, lupus (SLE), or an often very disabling condition called *scleroderma*, in which patients have arthritis and severe thickening of the skin, to the extent that they feel like a wax mannequin(369). Compared to patients with RA and yet another form of arthritis of the spine, called *ankylosing spondylitis* (AS), FM patients report pain that is greater in intensity, more likely to involve their arms, and more continuous; they also complain of more severe fatigue(370;371). Moreover, FM can occur in persons who already have one of these other conditions, like RA or lupus(372) (in other words, a single person can have RA and FM, or SLE and FM), and this may significantly worsen the quality of their life above and beyond what the RA or SLE does.

Some patients with FM develop disability that is considered severe enough to prevent them from seeking, continuing, or resuming gainful employment(58). Evidence supporting this comes from several sources and countries. For example, a survey of rheumatology clinics at six different centers across the U.S. revealed that 25% of FM patients were receiving some form of disability compensation(373). A survey of Canadian insurance company records found that FM was responsible for 9% of all disability payments, accounting for an estimated $200 million annually(374). In a study of Swedish patients with FM, 24% were receiving pensions(375). And in Britain, 50% of FM patients followed in a clinic stopped working because of their illness during the four years that they were being followed(376). In Norway, FM has been the most frequent single diagnosis for disability pensions(377).

In addition, lest critics say that disability rates are bound to be high in those being followed by specialists, because such patients are specifically seeking support for their disability claims, fibromyalgia is associated with high rates of disability not only in clinic populations, but in the general population as well, even among those not being seen by a specialist(198).

Because it is common and associated both with high rates of disability and increased use of health services, FM also exerts a huge economic impact upon society. In Canada, an estimated 700,000 Canadian adults have FM(378) resulting in $350 million in direct health care costs(379) and $200 million in private insurance costs annually(374). Per person FM-related costs in the U.S. may be several times higher(380), so that the direct and indirect costs of illness are in the billions of dollars.

2. Implications of a trauma-FM association

Prevention and Treatment: Despite numerous clinical trials involving a wide variety of medications, therapies, and programs, no treatment of FM, to date, can cure it, and many patients continue to have considerable pain, fatigue, and other ongoing symptoms(381). One potential reason for this is that FM patients who actually make it into a clinical trial may be particularly treatment-resistant. And one reason for this might be that it takes several years for the average person with FM to be referred to a doctor who has any form of expertise treating it. The average duration of symptoms among subjects in FM clinical trials often has exceeded five years(382-387). In general population surveys, the average duration of symptoms prior to diagnosis has been as long as 10 years or more(122;197). In other words, in the general population, the average person with FM has had their pain, fatigue, and other symptoms for 10 years or more before any doctor explains to them what they have.

If patients become less responsive to treatment the longer they have FM, the flip side to this is that being diagnosed earlier might result in better responses to treatment. If, for instance, some cases of FM stem from a recent injury, identifying those individuals early might improve their chances for a better outcome (e.g., less pain).

Trauma and medico-legal issues: One common reason FM patients come to see a rheumatologist, rehabilitation specialist, or some other 'expert' is for a disability assessment, a process which is both tedious and flawed. To date, there is no proven way to measure another person's level of disability, no matter what the suspected cause(58;388;389).

One of the most contentious issues in this setting is whether or not the FM was caused by an injury, either in the workplace or elsewhere. The role of the workplace injury becomes important if compensation for time off of work is being sought. In the mid 1980s, for example, a relative epidemic of repetitive strain injury (RSI) of the arms (especially carpal tunnel syndrome) occurred among telephone and key board operators working for Telecom Australia, resulting in a marked increase in compensation claims, litigation proceedings, and insurer expenses(390-395).

Motor vehicle related injuries are another common setting in which FM patients fight for long-term disability pensions and/or other compensation. In many jurisdictions in Canada and the U.S., chronic pain is deemed compensable by private or public insurers, but only if the pain clearly was precipitated by an injury. Insurers do not usually accept that chronic (long-term) widespread pain can be caused by an acute (sudden) localized injury. Many physicians feel that the role of the injury in chronic, widespread pain is less than the role of the injured person's personality, attitudes, and baseline level of medical and psychological health(396); taken to the extreme, this belief translates into only chronic 'complainers' or those who already were feeble getting long-term widespread pain after a sudden localized injury.

One author has argued that the diagnosis of FM should not be made at all in the medicolegal setting, both because of the ability of the FM patient to manipulate the tender point examination, and because of escalating compensation claims and costs related to this disorder(60;62;373). The next chapter will address these last two concerns.

3. Evidence supporting an association between trauma and FM

The strongest evidence supporting an association between trauma and FM is a relatively recently-published Israeli study by Buskila and colleagues, in which 22 (21.6%) of 102 adults with neck injuries developed FM within one year of their injury, compared to only one of 59 adults with lower extremity fractures (p = 0.001)(135). All subjects were recruited after presenting to an occupational medicine clinic for their injuries. It is of interest in Buskila's study that all 22 FM cases continued to work, a finding which is inconsistent with the high rates of disability in post-traumatic FM cases reported by others(18;359). But no mention is made as to whether they worked full or part time, or whether or not special accommodations were made for them.

143

One criticism of the Israeli study design has been that a pre-injury diagnosis of FM was not ruled out by examination for tender points, even though none of the 102 participating subjects had reported chronic pain prior to the injury. This criticism is unfounded, however, because the incidence of 21.6% is far too high to explain on the basis of pre-injury FM. First, the prevalence of FM has never exceeded 5% in any general population study, except in relatively narrow population subsets, like women between the ages of 55 and 64 in London Ontario(13;323), and women between the ages of 20 and 49 in the Norwegian city of Arendal(128), where it was as high as 10% in certain age groups. Second, the Israeli study population was largely male (65% and 73% in the two groups), in whom FM generally is less common. Finally, unless FM itself predisposes an individual to trauma, the pre-trauma prevalence of FM should have been the same in the two groups (the car accident and leg fracture groups), especially since the groups were similar in age and other characteristics.

A second criticism pertains to the study's ability to capture or identify everyone who has had a neck injury, since many individuals with a minor injury may not have sought health care services (again, by *capturing all neck injuries*, I mean being able to assess all those who have had a neck injury within the population of interest). Depending upon the number of such individuals, the estimate of FM incidence in those with neck injuries could drop significantly. However, it would require in excess of one thousand non-captured neck-injured individuals, and a capture rate of less than 10% (meaning that more than 90% of those who injured their neck were missed and not assessed to see whether or not they developed FM) to reduce the incidence estimate in the neck injury group to the same level as the lower extremity fracture group, both of which are highly unlikely.

A third criticism relates to an inherent bias in making the diagnosis of FM in individuals with neck injuries, given that 10 of the 18 FM tender points specified by the 1990 ACR criteria are in the neck and shoulder girdle area, and it was a difference in tender point count above the waist that distinguished the two Israeli groups(397). However, in

144

addition to having 11 or more tender points, all 22 FM cases in this study reported widespread pain, in accordance with the first ACR criterion. Moreover, three years later, 70 percent of the 20 patients available for follow-up still met the criteria for FM and had widespread pain, including all eleven women among the original 22 cases, leading the researchers to suggest that women were particularly prone to FM following a whiplash injury to the neck(398).

The 21.6% FM incidence figure does approximate the percentages, reported by Radanov (16%) and by Borchgrevink (18%), of individuals with persistent pain and other symptoms (including fatigue and sleep disturbances) two years after a whiplash injury(399;400). In the latter study, 16% still reported chronic pain and being "in a bad state of health" 15 years after their injury(399). Two other studies reported pain past one year in 3%(401) and 11%(402) of whiplash patients. Future post-traumatic FM incidence studies will need to follow and report on patient outcomes past one year, so as to estimate the natural history of and rate of remission in FM cases.

In a second case-control study performed by Al-Allaf and colleagues in the UK, those with new-onset FM were more than 60% more likely to report some significant trauma in the six months preceding the onset of their symptoms than those without FM(403).

Currently, no other published studies document an association between trauma and FM; and in Israel, another group of investigators failed to identify any association(404). Moreover, in two consecutive studies done in Lithuania, where the researchers claimed that knowledge of whiplash and compensation for whiplash were limited, no difference was found in the percentage of individuals with headaches, frequent headaches, or neck pain between those who had been in a rear-end motor vehicle collision, and those who had not(405-407). The main problems with these studies are that (1) the first study was done by asking people to recall an accident that happened 1 to 3 years earlier, and how they felt back then; (2) both studies involved almost exclusively males, because 90% of survey respondents were drivers; (3) they did not assess for pain elsewhere; and (4) no subject was assessed in person (everything was done via a mailed questionnaire). Consequently, whether an association exists or not remains unproven; and further research clearly is necessary.

These limitations aside, several studies provide at least a hypothetical construct for such an association(408). These include studies on: (1) sleep abnormalities after an injury; (2) local injury sites as a source of chronic distant regional pain; and (3) the concept of neuroplasticity, which will be defined later in this chapter.

Effects of Trauma on Sleep

In 1975, Harvey Moldofsky and Hugh Smythe reported detecting an association between pain and sleep disturbance in patients with chronic widespread pain and fatigue. Besides describing light or restless sleep and fatigue, these patients were found to have abnormal alpha wave interference particularly in Stage 4 non-rapid eye movement (non-REM) sleep, a pattern not observed in individuals who did not have pain and were otherwise healthy(104)[F]. Moreover, individuals who had suffered an emotionally distressing event (like trauma) at the onset of symptoms frequently had increased tenderness, and reported increased pain and stiffness upon awakening. Comparing two groups of healthy, non-athletic volunteers, Moldofsky and Scarisbrick noted diffuse pain and muscle tenderness in individuals deprived of Stage 4 non-REM, but not REM sleep; and, as in the prior study, muscle pain and tenderness increased overnight. It was hypothesized that Stage 4 sleep deprivation was important in the development of FM.

Subsequently, Moldofsky and his associates identified the same non-REM sleep disorder in women with chronic, widespread pain and fatigue who had suffered whiplash injuries of the neck as in women with FM and no history of injury(409). Although both groups reported symptoms of depression and anxiety, subsequent research failed to show the same sleep anomaly in women with depression alone(410). Moldofsky initially hypothesized that emotional distress caused by the traumatic event might result in

---

[F] This is covered in much greater detail in Chapter 10.

disturbed sleep, in turn resulting in the symptoms of FM(411). A further hypothetical link could be related to the effect of sleep deprivation on the normal night-time surge of growth hormone in the blood, given that: (A) slow-wave (i.e., delta wave) sleep deprivation abolishes the normal surge in night-time growth hormone levels(288), (B) levels of *somatomedin-C*, a hormone now more commonly called *insulin-like growth factor 1* (ILGF-1) that is closely linked to growth hormone, are low in FM patients(246), and (C) FM patients with low serum levels of somatomedin-C seem to have less pain when treated with growth hormone injections(287).

Local Injury Sites as a Source of Distant Regional Pain

The concept of chronic pain originating in muscles first appeared in the German medical literature in the mid to late nineteenth century. In those reports, pain was thought to be related to focal areas of *Muskelharten* (muscle hardness)(96;97) or *Muskelschwiele* (muscle calluses)(311) that the examiner could feel, and which were very tender.

In the 1930s, the concept that widespread pain could originate deep within muscle was supported by several studies by the two researchers, Kellgren and Lewis(6-9). Using blindfolded volunteers, they demonstrated that injecting saline (salt water) into muscles and tendons could result in pain that radiated out from the injection site to distant parts of the body. The distribution of the radiated pain caused by injecting a specific site was consistent from person to person; in other words, if you injected 10 different people all in the same spot, they all reported the pain spreading out in the same direction and covering roughly the same area. In 1950, another research team led by a Dr. Hardy reported that pain and tenderness could be produced in the abdomen (belly) and chest by injecting saline into ligaments in the spine(412).

More recently in Australia, researchers studied whiplash patients and identified small fractures involving small joints in the neck. As with the injections by Kellgren and Lewis, and later Hardy, these sites were associated with characteristic distributions of referred pain, including pain extending into the head, the shoulder area, and the arms(413;414).

Moreover, in a study in which patients were randomly assigned to one treatment group versus the other and not informed about which treatment they received until the study was over (we call this a *randomized, blinded clinical trial*), 24 patients who had chronic whiplash pain after a motor vehicle collision (MVC) were treated either with something called a *radiofrequency neurotomy* (basically a nerve block) or a mock (fake) treatment directed at those neck levels predicted to be the source of the pain. The average duration of pain relief was 263 days for subjects in the neurotomy group compared to just eigth days in the control group(415), a difference that was highly statistically significant, suggesting that these small joints in the neck actually were the cause of the pain, not just in the neck, but elsewhere as well. Interestingly, the same researchers, as part of their study protocol, administered a questionnaire called the Symptom Checklist 90 (SCL-90) both before and after treatment. Before the neurotomy or mock treatment, all the patients demonstrated very high levels of depression, obsessive-compulsion, anxiety, and other indicators of psychological distress. However, in those who actually received the neurotomy (as opposed to the mock or fake treatment), these values dropped significantly after the procedure, suggesting that the patients' high levels of psychological distress were caused by the pain, rather than the reverse(416).

Whereas the Australian research group generally focused upon two levels of the cervical spine (neck) -- C_{2-3} and C_{5-6} -- a Canadian researcher named Hugh Smythe has presented data to suggest that the C_{5-6} and the C_{6-7} levels are important sources of chronic, regional pain, and may be an important cause of FM(417;418). Both Smythe and others(395) have noted the presence of marked tenderness at specific areas that are some distance from the site of pain, sites that also are associated with reduced pain thresholds compared to the actual site of pain. All of this research supports the concept that widespread pain may be referred from a small focus of injury that often is not identifiable by standard imaging techniques, like X-rays, CAT scans, or MRIs. The neck appears to be a common source of chronic, referred pain; pain that may be relatively widespread. Smythe further argues that the lumbosacral spine (in the low back) and the

148

sacroiliac joints (in the buttock area) may be responsible for the lower extremity pain experienced by FM patients(29).

Trauma, Neuroplasticity and Chronic Pain

In 1950, Hardy and his research associates hypothesized that there are two types of pain sensitivity: (A) *primary pain sensitivity* (or *allodynia*) that involves increased sensitivity at the site of an injury, caused by local inflammation and direct nerve stimulation; and (B) *secondary pain sensitivity* that involves increased sensitivity extending beyond the site of injury, sometimes to remote sites some ways distant from the site of injury, caused by changes occurring within the brain and spinal cord(412). In 1991, a researcher named Zimmerman described a possible way by which injury to a nerve might initiate a complex interaction between these two forms of pain sensitivity, which eventually could lead to FM(419). A large body of evidence now supports the concept that pain can spread from injured to non-injured tissue by activation of various nerve processes in the brain, and that this distant pain can become both widespread and chronic, even persisting long after the initial injury has healed(420). This concept has been termed *neuroplasticity*(420).

A common example of referred pain from injured to non-injured tissue is the chest pain that accompanies a heart attack, which can be referred to sites as distant as the patient's hand, jaw, and ear(421). Phantom limb pain also may be caused by central neural activation, which means that the brain and spinal cord are permanently turned on by some injury that stimulates a distant nerve; for example, in one of the limbs(299). Memories of past pain also occur in patients who have had nerves torn completely apart at the level of the spinal cord, for example during motorcycle accidents and with direct spinal cord injuries (127).

Think about it: how could this possibly happen? How can someone have pain in their toes when their entire leg is gone; or when all nerves to the foot have been cut or torn away? Here's where a picture can be as good as a thousand words. Suppose, for instance, that someone suffers such a severe crush injury to their lower leg and foot (maybe they become crushed under debris when a building collapses during an earthquake), that the leg has to be amputated at the knee. Presumably, the leg and foot hurt terribly prior to being amputated. Consequently, those nerves bringing the sensation of pain back to the spinal cord (and, from there, the brain) were activated. In the first picture, below, note how, before amputation, the tissue below the knee has been injured and the nerve activated along its entire length. Now, in the second picture, note that, though the lower leg and foot are gone, the nerves that brought sensation back from the leg and foot are only partially gone; the parts that extend from the spinal cord to the knee still are there.

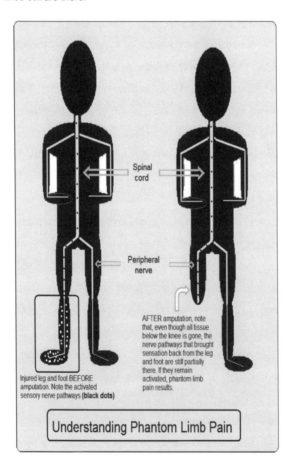

If, then, that length of nerve from the spinal cord to the knee still 'remembers' the pain that was in the foot, the person still will feel the pain, despite the foot being gone. In fact, if they look away or close their eyes, they might perceive the foot still to be there, feeling the pain in the exact location their foot would be, if it hadn't already been amputated.

Now, picture that the pain-activation changes in these nerves don't revert back to normal. THIS is what the theory of neuroplasticity is about. Is there research to support this? The answer is: unquestionably, starting with various studies in animals.

Several studies in animals have demonstrated the spread of pain from injured to non-injured tissue via the activation of what are called *central neural (nerve) pathways* (422;423). Perhaps the most striking model involved rats with experimentally-induced chemical burns to one paw. In these rats, even after all their nerves were cut, the rats continued to chew their burned paw to the point of chewing it off entirely(424). What this suggests is that the rats still felt the pain of the burn that occurred before their nerves all were cut, but none of the pain (from chewing) that occurred after their nerves were cut. This pain persisted even after complete surgical interruption of all nerve input from the injured area(425).

Also, an author and researcher named Mense has noted in rats that persistent muscle pain (that was caused experimentally) results in the expansion of particular types of nerves in the spinal cord (called *dorsal horn neurons;* note that the word *neuron* means *nerve cell*), indicating that the number of nerves that are irritated can increase over time(426). It is possible in humans that this spread of sensory activation to nearby nerve populations in the dorsal horn of the spine may result in injured individuals feeling that their pain is spreading which, in turn, might account for the development of FM following a localized injury (for example, whiplash) .

In addition, it has been shown that applying some noxious stimulus to a muscle (like a saline [saline = salt water] injection) causes the release of neurotransmitters (remember from an earlier chapter that neurotransmitters are to a nerve somewhat like what trains are to a train track) in the spine. The most likely transmitter is substance P, which has been demonstrated in nerves supplying sensation to muscles(427). Mense noted that, in experiments in which substance P has been administered in high concentrations in the dorsal horn of the spine, activation of pain neurons occurs at low concentrations, leading to long-lasting changes (depolarization) in nerve cell membranes(428;429). Contrary to other neurotransmitters, substance P spreads (diffuses) over long distances in the spinal cord after it is released. In this way, substance P is considered to be a *volume neurotransmitter*, meaning that it is capable of influencing large populations of nerve cells in the vicinity of where it initially was released(430). This property may be relevant in the spread of pain in humans. Moreover, substance P is not the only neuro-transmitter that can do this (128).

There are a number of changes demonstrated in FM that are strongly suggestive of *neuroplasticity*. These have been summarized in a very well-written paper by Dr. I. J. Russell(431). In three studies, FM patients have been found to have very high levels of substance P in their spinal fluid, compared to controls(74;208;432). Such high levels of substance P have been demonstrated both in patients with insidious onset and post-traumatic FM. Also, the neurotransmitter serotonin is known to inhibit the release of substance P, and FM patients have low levels of serotonin and related chemicals in spinal fluid (137).

Weigent and his research associates have proposed a hypothetical model for post-traumatic FM, which begins with muscle micro-trauma (small tears in the muscle that cannot be seen on CAT scan or MRI)(433). This is followed by increased pain transmission to the dorsal horn neurons in the spine. There, certain N-methyl-D-aspartate receptor sites in these nerve cells become activated by excitatory amino acids, substance P, and other chemicals like nerve growth factor, calcitonin gene-related peptide, and dynorphin, causing functional changes in the dorsal horn neurons and subsequent increased pain transmission to the brain(433).

Further research is necessary to test the various components of this and other models for FM. However, it is safe to say that considerable research evidence exists to support a role of recent injury as a cause of fibromyalgia.

Evidence against any association between trauma and FM

Critics offer four primary arguments against there being any association between trauma and FM. They are:

(A) FM does not exist;

(B) FM is a psychological, rather than a physical disease;

(C) There is inadequate proof of any association between trauma and FM; and

(D) Other factors are more important than the injury in determining chronic symptoms following an acute injury.

Reviewing chapters 4 through 15 of this book should eliminate any concern you have regarding the first two objections; and reviewing what I have written so far in this chapter should largely counter the third. Let me focus then on the fourth argument against trauma as a cause of FM.

Are other factors more important than the trauma as the cause of FM?

The two factors that generally are ascribed by critics of any trauma-FM association as being more important than the injury are: (1) the patient's baseline personality traits and psychological status; and (2) whether or not litigation (the legal system) is involved.

Personality and Psychological Factors: As stated earlier, many physicians across different medical specialties feel that the role of the injury in chronic, widespread pain is less than the role of other factors, including the injured person's personality, attitudes, and baseline level of medical and psychological health(396) To date, there are no studies reporting predictors of outcome in FM.

There are, however, studies that have looked at predictors of outcome in whiplash injuries and low back pain. Many of these studies are methodologically weak. For example, in a look back at 1,551 whiplash patients in the province of Quebec, several patient factors were found to be independent predictors of outcome(401). However, the primary outcome was termination of compensation payments, rather than documented improvement in symptoms; and it is possible that a large number of individuals had benefits terminated irrespective of how well or poorly they were feeling; hence, it is inappropriate to assume that termination of benefits is an accurate indicator of clinical recovery.

A Swiss study found three crash-related factors, as opposed to only two pre-injury variables, to be predictors of outcome in 137 whiplash patients(434;435). However, subjects were recruited non-randomly and from two divergent and possibly non-representative sources: 117 referred from a family practice, and 16 'chosen' from the regional agency of a Swiss accident insurance company. More importantly, the analysis included a complicated statistical test called *logistic regression*, apparently including 62 baseline characteristics. Speaking as a statistician[G], I can assure you that their sample size was far too small to test that number of variables. To adequately assess 62 different variables in a logistic regression model, they would have needed five to ten times as many patients as they had.

In a survey of 50 consecutive patients presenting for emergency services following a rear-end car accident, psychological status at 3 months, but not one week after the injury was predictive of long term outcome(436). In another prospective survey of 88 neck sprain patients injured in car accidents, in which psychological profile was measured when the patients first saw a doctor, pre-injury personality traits were not found to predict outcome(437).

In a study of 116 patients seeing a family physician for acute low back pain, a pre-injury history of anxiety or depression was the best predictor of disability; however, follow-up

---

[G] In addition to my medical degree (MD), I have a PhD in Epidemiology and Biostatistics.

154

was limited to six weeks(438). Other studies on chronic low back pain not necessarily associated with injury have noted that psycho-social variables appear to be important in long-term outcomes(439;440). However, psychological status usually was measured after more than six months of symptoms, so no baseline assessments were available.

In summary then:

There is no convincing scientific evidence that someone's baseline personality or psychological status predicts whether or not they will develop FM or chronic pain after an injury.

Litigation: Many also feel that litigation (suing for disability payments or compensation) plays a significant part in chronic post-traumatic pain and FM. An Alberta judge has characterized FM "as a court-driven ailment that has mushroomed into big business for plaintiffs"(115). High annual insurance costs in Canada support this assertion(374). As mentioned earlier, in a recent survey in Lithuania, where compensation for traumatic injuries generally is not available, drivers involved in rear-end car collisions one to three years earlier were no more likely to report neck pain or headache (35% and 53%, respectively) than age- and sex-matched controls with no prior history of a car crash (30% and 50%, respectively)(441). Chronic headache and neck pain, defined as symptoms at least seven days per month, also were no more common in the car accident (8.4% and 9.4%, respectively) versus control group (6.9% and 5.9%, respectively). However, significant limitations to the study include the disproportionate number of male subjects (78%), the exclusion of motor vehicle passengers, and the later, non-random inclusion of 30 female passengers to the car accident group, because the researchers felt that there was an inadequate number of female drivers in the study. In other words, the study was very poorly done.

Some have argued that legislation negating whiplash(442) and repetitive strain injuries

(RSI) (390-395) as compensable conditions was responsible for a fall in insurance claims in Australia in the late 1980s. However, the same authors admit that there had been a fall in insurance claims prior to legislation and that other factors, such as legislation requiring the use of seat belts, may have contributed significantly to the decrease in claims. Moreover, using the number of claims to represent the number of cases of disease is subject to significant bias, because legislation refusing claims almost certainly results in the under-reporting of cases. Also, that FM appears to be more prevalent in less-developed countries argues against litigation having a major role in disease prevalence(19). Finally, at least two recent studies on whiplash patients, in which patients were followed long-term after their injury, have demonstrated that the role of litigation on outcome is minimal(443;444).

The two questions posed at the beginning of this chapter – (1) Does an association exist between trauma and FM? and (2) What might such an association mean? - have not been answered with 100% certainty. But, to be fair, relatively few questions in medicine ever are. What can be said is:

1. That an association very likely does exist;

2. That FM after trauma likely is caused by changes in sleep, the spine, spinal cord and brain, including changes in neurotransmitters and in the nerves themselves; and

3. That the balance of evidence already in existence supports some cases of FM being caused by an injury, especially injuries of the neck and lower spine.

CHAPTER 17

FIBROMYALGIA AND DISABILITY

As stated in the previous chapter, it is not uncommon for someone with FM to have symptoms severe enough that they become unable to work, either full-time or at all (58;445); and many of these people find themselves applying for some sort of disability payments, either short-term or long-term. In addition, a sizeable percentage of these patients will have suffered an injury, so that they are applying for compensation. In the case of a car accident (for example, a whiplash injury, as described in the previous chapter), they may be taking the other driver to court. In those with a work-related injury, they may be suing their employer. In all these instances, an adversarial relationship may develop (i.e., they end up fighting someone else for money). The fight may be long and bitter. And, because FM is less accepted than many other disabling conditions or injuries, 'proving' disability becomes even more difficult.

People with FM experience health and financial losses that are similar in degree to those of patients with rheumatoid arthritis(446). Rates of actual inability to work among those with FM, whether seen in a clinic or assessed in the general community, generally range between about 25% and 50%(198;373;375;376), meaning that between one in four, and one half of all those with FM claim to be unable to work, at least full time. Many such individuals are successful having their disability recognized, with FM among the most common reasons for a disability pension to be awarded in Canada(374), Norway(377), and elsewhere. This is true despite the fact that there is so much resistance against both FM's validity and its potential for 'true' disability (26;27;76;77;85;91;98;111-113;115;200;328;329;360).

The arguments against FM being a legitimate source of disability are much the same as the ones that already have been countered over the course of this book, and which were listed and explained in greater detail in Chapter 3. Again, the most common arguments against FM are:

1. Fibromyalgia is just the usual aches and pains everyone has, expressed in people who can't deal with them.

2. Fibromyalgia is a syndrome, not a disease.

3. Fibromyalgia only exists because of today's politically-correct bleeding-heart society.

4. Fibromyalgia only exists because of an overly-generous compensation system.

5. Fibromyalgia only exists because some people are lazy and want society to take care of them.

6. Fibromyalgia only exists because some doctors and researchers profit from its so-called 'existence'.

7. The way fibromyalgia is diagnosed is inherently flawed.

8. The way fibromyalgia initially was defined is inherently flawed.

9. All the symptoms of fibromyalgia are subjective.

10. Fibromyalgia is 100% subjective; there are no objective physical findings to suggest the disease is real.

11. There is no anatomical or physiological basis for fibromyalgia.

12. None of the objective physical or physiological findings in fibromyalgia are specific to this disorder.

13. No one has fibromyalgia until they are told they have it; if you removed the fibromyalgia label, these people wouldn't be nearly as 'sick'.

14. Fibromyalgia is a psychological, and not a physical disease.

As these arguments have all been countered thoroughly in earlier chapters, I will not do it here. Instead, let me focus on arguments specifically relating to assessing disability in someone with FM. They are:

1. There is no way to objectively assess the level of disability in someone with FM.

2. Even if FM is real, the individual patient can 'fake' it, and also fake being

disabled.

3. All the patient needs is some work-hardening program to return to work.

Argument #1: There's no way to objectively assess disability in FM

To begin with, it is important to understand the complexity of assessing anyone with disability? One issue that complicates things from the outset is that insurance policies differ widely. For example, some clauses state that someone is disabled so long as they are unable to return to their former occupation or job, or something appropriate to their level of training. In other words, a brain surgeon or lawyer or Nobel-winning physicist won't be forced to work at a fast food restaurant, just because he or she 'can'. Meanwhile, other policies define disabled as being unable to work at 'any job'. Think about this for a second. There are security jobs where one's primary function is sitting in a chair watching a screen or monitor (or several). Theoretically, you could place a quadriplegic individual in their chair in front of one of these monitors, and rig up some voice-activated system for them to sound an alarm. As long as they had a mobile partner who could take care of everything else, wouldn't they be able to work? The answer is... okaaay. I guess so. But who actually would subject someone to this, unless the person himself or herself truly wanted to do it?

This comes down to the second more important question than 'can this person work?' This question is: is this person employable'? This is an ENTIRELY different question. In essence, the question is: given the current job market and available competition, is there a reasonable probability that someone will be willing to hire this person, and continue to employ them, knowing their limitations? Again, this is a much different question than *can they work*?

I once asked the following question to another doctor who always (and I mean ALWAYS) refused to accept a patient being disabled; the question was: "Okay Doc...

will YOU hire them?" In that particular instance, the disabled person was a former receptionist with FM, and the doctor in question just happened to need a new receptionist. Interestingly, he didn't even attempt to answer my question.

Another question that complicates the disability assessment is: can this person work at all? For example, some patients are seeking or are offered partial disability pensions, usually expressed as a percentage. For example, someone who is paralyzed in one arm following a motorcycle accident might be awarded 30% disability, meaning that they will be given just 30% of what their full disability payments would be, under the assumption that they still could do something to make up the difference. So, assessing disability is not just proving that someone is disabled. One also must consider how disabled. Can they return to their own job part-time? To any job? Are they 20% disabled? 50% disabled? 3% disabled? And, most importantly, are they actually employable?

It is, at best, confusing.

How can you truly say if someone with FM is disabled and, if so, how much? These are good questions. However, they are not questions that should be reserved for those with FM. How, for example, does one assess the level of disability in someone with rheumatoid arthritis, or lupus, or multiple sclerosis, or a long list of other non-controversial disorders? In some, it is easy. In an RA patient who has grossly swollen joints and obvious joint deformities, it may not be that difficult; and the same is true of a patient with lupus who has something called *lupus cerebritis* (inflammation of the brain), which can be documented on MRI and often leads to the patient being grossly confused, psychotic or even comatose; and it is true of the MS patient who is diffusely paralyzed. But what about patients with RA, lupus or MS who are not so obviously disabled? Fatigue, for example, can be a highly disabling symptom in all these patients, being the most commonly reported serious health issue by patients with lupus, claimed by 87%; interestingly, this is the exact same percentage as those who, in the same study, reported being unable to perform previous activities(447). So... how do you rate another person's fatigue?

160

Come to think of it... how do rate the nausea of someone receiving chemotherapy for cancer? Or their weakness, which is more a lack of endurance than true weakness? And if you can't rate these things, why can't patients with cancer receiving chemotherapy all work? Would FM critics who use the 'FM symptoms are subjective' argument want them all to work too? I certainly hope not.

How do you rate the stiffness of the person with RA or lupus if they don't have gross joint swelling; or of someone with polymyalgia rheumatic (PMR), who likely won't have ANY physical findings?

The list goes on.

Various assessment questionnaires have been developed, on which patients with various forms of arthritis rate their own function. Commonly used examples of these are the Health Assessment Questionnaire (HAQ)(448), the HAQ Disability Index (HAQ-DI)(449), and the Arthritis Impact Measurement Scale (AIMS)(450;451). However, these questionnaires all rely on patients themselves rating their performance in various household activities and tasks (so all the answers are subjective, not objective); and none of these tools was designed to look at work disability, per se. For example, there is a big difference between being able to dress yourself or stand up from a straight chair and being able to work full time. On the HAQ- and the HAQ-DI, the closest you get to assessing work ability are the items asking patients if they can run errands and shop or do chores such as vacuuming or yard work(452); but the questions only ask about one's level of difficulty doing these tasks, and not how long they can do it, or how regularly, or how long it takes them to complete the task. Again, puttering around in the garden for an hour three days a week on your own schedule is much different than getting up and being ready to work at an appointed time, travelling to and from work, and putting in 8-hour shifts five or so days per week. And who really would hire someone who takes two to three times as long as anyone else to do a given job?

Much the same can be said of the Fibromyalgia Impact Questionnaire (FIQ)(453), and of the 42-item Fibromyalgia Checklist (FC-42) that my research colleagues and I developed and tested(197), the former asking patients to rate the level of a variety of symptoms (like pain and fatigue), and rate their level of difficulty with certain personal and household tasks, which range from climbing stairs and making a bed to going shopping and doing yard work(453;454). Actual copies of the HAQ and FIQ, the two most commonly used questionnaires, can be downloaded from http://aramis.stanford.edu/downloads/HAQ%20-%20DI%202007.pdf and http://www.drlowe.com/clincare/clinicalforms/fiq.pdf, respectively.

Another issue here is that the same symptom or the same level of symptom severity that is disabling to one person might not be to another. Would you really want a truck driver on the road who complains of disabling fatigue? And I have a brother who is a classical pianist. To him, a permanent injury to one finger likely would end his career; but not so for a truck driver, or a receptionist, or a radio announcer, or most people. On the other hand, some quadriplegics do work... a very small percentage, perhaps, but Stephen Hawking and the late Christopher Reeve come to mind. But the circumstances of this world-renowned scientist and equally-famous actor must be considered entirely different. Both would have had bountiful financial resources to access the best support systems available; and who wouldn't do everything they could to help these two great and highly-influential men to continue to contribute? Consequently, these two famous quadriplegics cannot possibly be compared to the person with a grade-10 education who was previously working in a factory or a store; or the single mother who has been doing her best to support her family working nights. How are they going to pay for the resources available to people like Hawking and Reeve; and what employer or agency is going to bend over backwards to accommodate them?

My main points are:
1. There is no way to objectively rate the severity of most symptoms, regardless of the person's condition, since all symptoms are, by definition, subjective(90). To single out FM patients and say that they don't deserve disability or compensation

payments because you can't 'objectively' determine their level of ability and disability is (1) grossly unjust; and (2) not supported by any research in the scientific literature.

2. Many other factors come into play, like the type of policy the person has; the person's education, experience, influence, and level and breadth of training; the person's age; the job market; the nature, number, and severity of symptoms and their potential affect upon the specific job or jobs being considered; and others. And, again, this applies to almost all individuals applying for disability or compensation, whether they have FM, lupus, RA, MS or whatever. To believe otherwise is just prejudiced.

Argument #2: FM and FM-related disability can be faked

This argument actually is just another way of phrasing the first argument. In other words, since disability in FM can't be objectively determined, it can be faked. The counter-arguments to this essentially are the same as those just stated. If disability can be faked by a person with FM, it also can be faked by patients with a whole host of other conditions. Again, unless the RA patient has grossly swollen joints or deformities, and especially if 'all' he or she complains about are pain, fatigue, and stiffness, who's to say they aren't faking, or at least exaggerating? Ditto for lupus and PMR and the cancer patient receiving chemotherapy who says they feel weak and nauseated, and on and on. Do I think any of these cancer patients are faking? Frankly, I consider it heartless even to question them. How then, can anyone justify discrediting another person's pain, without compelling evidence contradicting it – like seeing them doing handstands and back-flips on their way into the office (again, I exaggerate a bit to make my point). And, even worse, how can someone even start to justify discrediting the hundreds of thousands (if not millions) of FM patients worldwide who claim to be disabled.

Remember again that there are a whole host of objective findings, both physical and chemical, in those with FM (please refer back to Chapters 10 through 13); we just don't routinely test for them. And, as mentioned in Chapter 11, in one study, a number of doctors were asked to examine several FM patients and also actors who had been instructed to fake having FM, and the doctors were able to accurately diagnose FM 80% of the time(79). Clearly, there are non-verbal clues that doctors can rely on to determine whether or not a given patient is attempting to deceive them. What is important is that the doctor is fair in his or her assessment. A well-trained, conscientious, and impartial physician should be able to see through most attempts at deception. Fibromyalgia critics may insist that this is exactly what they are doing. But how can anyone who insists upon ignoring the mountainous volume of scientific evidence that has been presented in this book while forming their opinions, possibly call themselves 'impartial'?

Also as stated earlier, in Chapter 11, some doctors use so called *control points* to detect those who are faking, believing that anyone who is tender everywhere and not just at the 18 FM tender points listed in the American College of Rheumatology (ACR) criteria must be faking. But the use of these points has been scientifically debunked, by at least five published scientific studies that demonstrated that FM patients are more tender not just at the 18 ACR criteria points, but everywhere(78-82), because of the abnormal way their nervous system processes and regulates pain. To use my tiger versus panther analogy again (Chapter 11), FM is a black panther, and NOT a tiger. It is the very nature of the disease that FM patients hurt and are tender almost everywhere, because the disease is not of the muscles themselves, but of the central nervous system. The disrupted way in which the FM patient's brain and nerves process potentially painful stimuli often causes them to have pain and tenderness anywhere and everywhere. In other words, FM is a black panther, and something like rheumatoid arthritis (RA) is a tiger. Like the tiger and panther share areas that are black, the patient with FM and the one with RA will have common areas of tenderness. But the FM patient also will be tender in areas where the RA patient is not, just like the black panther is black in areas where the tiger is not.

Once more quoting the prominent FM researcher Dr. Fred Wolfe(82): *"Control point positivity should not be used to disqualify a diagnosis of FM."*

Another way some doctors choose to identify those who are faking is by using something called *Waddell s signs*(455). These are a group of physical signs, first described in 1980 by Gordon Waddell and three associates, that were intended to identify a non-physical or psychological component to chronic low back pain. They include (1) tests to detect superficial and diffuse tenderness and/or non-anatomic tenderness; (2) simulation tests that are based on movements which produce pain, without actually causing that movement (for example, telling a patient that you are stretching their hamstring muscle without actually doing so); (3) distraction tests, which involve re-doing a previously positive test when the patient's attention is distracted (for example, is the person still tender over their shoulder when the doctor is moving it to check its range of movement); (4) assessments for localized weakness or sensory changes that are inconsistent with accepted neuroanatomy; and (5) looking for over-reactions, like a patient falling down and screaming when blown upon (admittedly, this is another extreme example to illustrate my point).

While these tests may seem useful, you must first recall that they were designed to detect malingering (faking) in patients with localized, low back pain, NOT in patients with the disrupted central pain mechanisms of FM. Second, at least three papers have been written demonstrating how these signs are not particularly sensitive or specific at ruling out true physical disease(456-458), one of these studies by Waddell himself(456). In the end, the conclusion of one group of authors was that there was "little evidence for the claims of an association between Waddell signs and secondary gain and malingering. The preponderance of the evidence points to the opposite: no association(458)."

And yet another way doctors performing medico-legal assessments sometimes discredit individual patients is by citing what they have seen in surveillance tapes, typically filmed by a private investigator who has been hired by the insurance company. I return to my earlier handstands and back-flips statement by saying, virtually never, having reviewed hundreds of these tapes, have I ever seen anything at all conclusive. Yes, I have seen patients coming outside to do light gardening in their front yard for maybe an hour – but these patients weren't claiming to be bedridden; and one hour of light gardening a few steps from your own home on a nice sunny day when you feel better than average does not equate with being able to return to work full-time, on a rigid time schedule, travelling miles to and from work in wind, rain, and snow. Similarly, in my mind, carrying four bags of groceries from one's car to the house after 20 minutes of grocery shopping hardly translates into being ready for full-time employment; unless, of course, the person was transporting full-sized hay bales for their horse. I also had one doctor vehemently argue that this one patient clearly was faking everything because she was seen leaving her house, driving 10 minutes downtown, running several errands, and then returning home… it turns out that it wasn't even the patient in question, but her younger sister, who regularly stopped by to help with things like this. And, best of all, the private investigator had been outside the house for about a week before catching ANY sign of the 'patient' leaving her home; what healthy person stays indoors like that?

The fact is that disability generally tends to be under-estimated, and not over-estimated, by physicians. In one study, for example, 118 doctors in both university-based and community-based medical practices, assessing 408 patients, failed to identify 68% of the legitimate sources of disability(459); this means that they averaged missing more than two disabled patients out of every three. These were patients with a wide range of underlying conditions, with likely only a smallish percentage having FM. Under-estimating disability may be particularly problematic in diseases involving the muscles and joints, where the interaction between function and job requirements strongly affects work performance(460). The researcher Liang and his colleagues, for example, compared the disability assessments of independent arthritis experts (rheumatologists) against the judgments of the U.S. Social Security Administration (SSA), and found that, where the two assessments were in agreement in 35 of 52 disability patients (which equals 67% of the claimants) with either RA, lupus or osteoarthritis, the experts also identified disability in eleven persons for whom the SSA rejected the disability claim (which equals 21% of the claimants, or roughly one in five)(461). Though no similar study has been done for FM, I strongly suspect that the numbers would be far worse for claimants, given inherent biases against FM.

Also, given the prolonged period of time that many patients often wait (sometimes years) before any payments are received, why would these people fake it for so long? Countless FM sufferers have lost their jobs, their incomes, their savings, their homes, their families, their social activities, their dreams, and so much else. Is it really worth it for all these people?

In other words – Yes, it may be possible for some signs and symptoms of FM to be exaggerated or faked. But:

1. Most patients with FM probably are NOT faking;

2. There is no evidence that any greater percentage of patients with FM are faking than with many other universally-accepted medical conditions;

3. So-called *fibromyalgia control points* and *Waddell's* signs are not useful at identifying those who are faking;

4. Surveillance tapes rarely provide any definitive evidence, and must always be viewed with an open mind and extreme caution;

5. In general, doctors tend to under-estimate rather than over-estimate disability;

6. A well-trained, conscientious and impartial physician should be able to see through most attempts at deception by taking a thorough medical history and performing an appropriate physical examination; and

167

7. Overall, I place my faith more in a patient's regular doctor and/or specialist(s), especially if they see the patient regularly and have been following them for some time, than in the opinions of any doctor who sees them once in such an artificial and potentially-biased setting as an independent medical evaluation, so long as the former doctor(s) is(are) conscientious, reasonably informed in the area of chronic pain, and open-minded.

Argument #3: All the patient needs is a good work-hardening program

Some doctors feel that FM patients just have gotten soft, perhaps aided by bleeding-heart physicians who have coddled them for too long(77;112). To support this, they point out various reports that document no inflammatory changes in muscle(100;101;272;273;462), but do show changes that <u>might</u> be signs of de-conditioning(100;101). The flip side to this, then, is that all such patients need is to be toughened up a bit. Hence, the birth and promotion of so-called *work-hardening programs*. Essentially, what such programs do is gradually re-introduce the sick or injured patient back into the work force, starting with maybe a couple of hours three days per week, and then slowly increasing the hours over weeks or months until the individuals finally are back to working full time. This might sound like a great idea to some FM critics, but for a few critical problems:

1. The entire concept misses the point; FM is NOT a disease of muscle dysfunction or de-conditioning. Instead, a growing mountain of evidence indicates that it is a disease of the central, peripheral and autonomic (involuntary) nervous systems, especially related to the processing of pain and regulation of blood flow;

2. Exercise often makes FM patients feel worse, especially in terms of their pain and fatigue;

3. Pain and muscle fatigue are NOT the only disabling symptoms of FM; and

168

4. The evidence that such programs work at all is limited and not very convincing; and there is none for individuals with post-traumatic pain and FM.

Recall, from Chapter 11, the large number of abnormal processes that are going on at both the brain and peripheral nerve levels in patients with FM. These changes affect brain blood flow, electrical activity, and metabolism(222-226;230;231;236;277;290;463-470), electrical activity in the brain during sleep(104;106;107;409;411;471), and the chemicals called *neurotransmitters* that help to transmit messages along and between nerves(74;208;211-214;216;217;247;289;468;472;473). Taken together, there is an overall disruption in the person's ability to turn pain on and off and regulate its severity in a normal way, leading to increased widespread pain and sensitivity, often even to light touch(226;238;411;419;431;465;474;475).

Note no mention of muscles here. So what sense, really, does it make to say that all these people need is to exercise and get their muscles used to working again? Think about this for a second more. When you are sick with a bad flu and feel so fatigued and achy all over, do you really think that getting up and out of bed and working out is the way to feel better, while still sick? Will the increased activity help your fever, or your cough, or your nausea and vomiting? Of course not, because you don't feel poorly just because your muscles are de-conditioned. You feel poorly because you have a virus that is wreaking havoc with your immune system, causing chemicals (called *cytokines*) to be released that cause your diffuse aching, fevers, fatigue, and everything else.

If we accept that FM is real, that it does not spontaneously get better, that it is NOT a disease of muscle, and that it is a condition associated with a large number of symptoms besides just muscle pain and fatigue, why should we assume that working out will make all the symptoms resolve? Would this work with multiple sclerosis, another disease of the nervous system? Of course not. That is not to say that a doctor wouldn't advise an MS patient whose disease is going into relative remission to slowly start exercising, or even to slowly and gradually return to work. But the patient must be entering into remission (in other words, their underlying disease must be improving) before the doctor encourages them to increase their activities again. Would we send a patient with rheumatoid arthritis and hugely swollen joints and morning stiffness lasting until the mid afternoon back to work before the swelling went down and the stiffness was dramatically improved? I hope not.

In truth, some studies have shown that multi-dimensional rehabilitation and/or behavioral programs do help patients with FM. Having said this, the benefits generally are slight and patients who are off work generally do not return to work following completion of these programs, at least not for some time(476). And none of these programs were designed specifically as return-to-work (RTW) programs.

Work-hardening RTW programs generally were designed to gradually return a person to work after an injury. Proponents(477) often cite a handful of older studies in which patients with either low back pain or whiplash injuries were gradually and successfully returned to work(478-480). However, each of the studies suffered from major methodological flaws. Catchlove and Cohen(478) looked back to compare the records (this type of study is called a *retrospective study*) of patients directed by the Worker's Compensation Board (WCB) of Ontario to participate in a return-to-work program, versus those who had not been referred to such a program. Not surprisingly, they found that 60% in the work-hardening group returned to work over the duration of treatment, compared to just 25% in the other group. But this is nothing more than one would expect, given that WCB most likely referred patients to the return-to-work (RTW) program who had been assessed as more likely to be successful. In other words, it almost certainly was the patients' baseline health status (level of pain and level of disability, etc., as described by the patient's own physician or physicians) that was predictive of their return to work, and not whether or not they participated in the RTW program. In addition, those entered into the RTW program may have felt coerced into returning to work, rather than feeling that they had a choice, so they accepted a greater level of pain than those not entered into the RTW program, who likely felt less pressure and waited until their symptoms had subsided more.

The two other studies were similar(479;480), in that those entered into the RTW program were compared against those who were not deemed suitable or otherwise were rejected from or themselves elected not to participate in the program. Why were some patients not entered into the program? Why did some refuse to participate? Perhaps, and quite likely, the non-participants were those with worse overall baseline levels of pain and other symptoms, so it would be expected that fewer of the non-treated group would re-enter the workforce over the duration of the study. And, again, pressure or lack of pressure to return to work may have played a factor, as well.

Finally, the patients in these studies all had a localized injury, and none were reported to have FM. Comparisons of FM patients randomly assigned to a RTW program versus those not randomly assigned to such a program have not been reported. Without them, any argument that this is the solution to returning FM patients to work is nothing more than one person's opinion.

So...

Can FM cause disability?

I think that the vast majority of evidence, much of which I have described in this book, indicates that it can; or, at the very least, we should have no more reason to doubt it than for a whole host of other universally-accepted conditions.

How should the FM patient be assessed for disability?

The answer to this is: in the same conscientious and impartial way that ALL physicians should assess ALL patients. Fibromyalgia patients deserve no more, but also no less than this.

CHAPTER 18

FIBROMYALGIA:

THE ANSWER IS BLOWIN' IN THE WIND

To finish off, here is the opinion paper that I wrote to start this all off. In retrospect, I think it represents the pinnacle of my professional career as a fibromyalgia researcher and clinician. It certainly has received the most attention. If you want the original manuscript, it can be found in the Journal of Rheumatology for the year 2004, in volume 31, on pages 636 through 639. Thanks go to the Journal of Rheumatology for allowing me to print it here.

■■

How many times can a man turn his head and pretend that he just doesn't see?

--Bob Dylan, 'Blowin' in the Wind'

These immortalized words have rung true repeatedly throughout the sordid history of humankind. Yet it should seem startling that Dylan's words might apply to physicians, who recite the Hippocratic Oath, and promise to ease pain and suffering and "do no harm." Nonetheless, these words too often do apply to physicians, perhaps no more frequently than when many such physicians are asked to deal with fibromyalgia (FM). For those unfortunate patients who suffer from FM, "Hippocratic" often rings more like "hypocritical." In desperation, patients turn to those learned in Medicine and professing to help them, only to hear their malady called — nothing at all: "an illusionary entity"(1), "a common non-entity"(2), "mass hysteria"(3),"the syndrome of feeling out of sorts"(4). Many in the medical profession have chastised FM, calling for "a return to common sense"(5) by discarding the label, and the concept, altogether. But why? And why are these comments so often laced with venom? Why are those who oppose the FM concept so verbal and destructive, many going out of their way to write position papers

173

about an area in which they have done no research, and seem so oblivious and impervious to the research of others?

The answer lies far beyond a lack of acceptance of a poorly understood and poorly treated entity. We have little understanding of disease mechanisms for many well accepted disorders, such as polymyalgia rheumatica, migraine headache, and trigeminal neuralgia. And we have very few effective treatments for disorders such as scleroderma and ankylosing spondylitis. Yet none of these disorders comes under the same intensely zealous scrutiny as FM.

What is it about FM that provokes such ire? It should not be that FM symptoms all are subjective — all symptoms are, by definition, subjective(6,7), irrespective of their setting. Whether caused by FM or cancer, tendonitis or ischemic heart disease, symptoms such as pain, fatigue, nausea, and dizziness cannot be measured objectively. We must rely on patient reports, then choose to believe them, or not.

Some have used objective evidence of tissue pathology, such as gross swelling or radiographic changes, as an objective proxy for pain; the corollary to this is that they believe that the absence of objectively measurable tissue pathology is an argument against the presence of "true pain." However, both halves of this reasoning are flawed. Medical practice abounds with disorders in which the degree of pain and degree of objective tissue pathology do not correlate: headache, migraine headache, trigeminal neuralgia, phantom limb pain, kidney stones, and the Charcot joint. We cannot and should not fool ourselves into believing that we can estimate another individual's pain. One day, technology capable of measuring the pain of others will exist, but it does not exist — at least for use in clinical practice — at the time of this writing. We all will have to wait.

No one can reasonably justify the zealous anti-FM movement by arguing that there are no objective physical findings among FM patients. First of all, there are many well accepted disorders that lack objective physical findings. The same physicians who have such difficulty understanding and accepting FM have no problems at all injecting or operating on patients with de Quervain's tenosynovitis, medial and lateral epicondylitis, rotator cuff tendonitis, and greater trochanteric bursitis, despite the utter absence of any 'objective' physical findings in any of these conditions. Tenderness, certainly, cannot be considered 'objective'. And yet, it is one of the mainstays of physical examination, be it of the teeth, the abdomen, the muscles, the joints, or elsewhere. Moreover, should we be any less believing when we identify tenderness on examination, than we should be when we identify alterations in sensation, cognition, or strength? Again, we badger our medical students on the importance of examining for all of these. Why? Why, indeed, if these 'non-objective' findings are not fit to be believed anyway?

Many FM patients do have measurable alterations in skin tissue compliance and reactive hyperemia, findings that are measurable and objective(8). FM naysayers pay no attention to this, perhaps claiming that these are non-specific findings that, further, many patients with FM do not have. And yet I have observed the same physicians enthusiastically gather around them a horde of medical students to demonstrate livedo reticularis as a sign of systemic lupus erythematosus (SLE).

The acidic reaction towards FM cannot be justified by arguing that there are no pathophysiologic changes in FM patients. To begin with, for years there has been a large and rapidly expanding body of scientific evidence demonstrating numerous pathophysiologic differences between FM patients and healthy controls. As early as the late 1970s, Moldofsky was reporting alterations in brain wave activity in Stage IV sleep, alterations found in other chronic pain states but not in dysthymia(9). These findings have been replicated many times over, and most recent research has found that alpha wave intrusion into Stage IV sleep is predictive of symptom severity(10). How possibly could FM research subjects manipulate these results? The answer is that they could not.

For more than 10 years, we have known of various hormonal and other biochemical changes such as abnormal diurnal variations in corticosteroid secretion(11), low serum

175

concentrations of somatomedin-C(12) and tryptophan(13), low cerebrospinal fluid (CSF) levels of 5-hydroxytryptophan(14), and high CSF levels of substance P(15). More recent research has provided a potential explanation for some of these findings, including reduced serum activity of prolylendopeptidase (a cytosolic endopeptidase responsible for the inactivation of a variety of algesic peptides, including substance P)(16).

Thermographically measured skin temperature appears to be lower in the back(17) and higher in the hands(18) in FM patients compared to healthy controls, implying some alteration in normal dermal sympathetic activity in FM. More recent research has shown further evidence of altered autonomic nerve function in response to orthostatic stress(19).

Two small recent studies suggest an alteration in the pattern of cerebral blood flow(20,21), which may help to explain the debilitating fatigue and cognitive difficulties described by these patients. The list of scientifically demonstrated physiologic abnormalities in FM patients goes on and on. Detailing them all is far beyond the scope of this editorial. Nonetheless, this research exists and no critic should verbalize his or her opinions without performing an educated and unbiased review of it. Through all this research, FM has become the prototype chronic, systemic pain disorder, much the way that SLE is the prototype chronic, systemic autoimmune disorder. Scientists who accept that we have much to learn about pain have learned much, much of this knowledge coming from studying FM. Such knowledge has been attained by reaching beyond the over-simplistic, grossly anatomic view of the world to which so many of us seem confined.

Some argue that these pathophysiologic irregularities are not specific for FM. But this, also, is not a valid argument against the acceptance of FM. If it were, we would be forced to question the validity of an almost endless number of otherwise well-accepted disorders for which all pathophysiologic changes are non-specific. Foremost among these would be SLE. The positive predictive value of the detection of antinuclear antibodies (ANA) is no greater than one percent, which makes the testing for ANA 50 times less predictive than the flip of a coin. In addition, not one of the many other pathophysiologic abnormalities of SLE is specific to SLE. Does SLE not exist? How about rheumatoid arthritis (RA)? Polymyalgia rheumatica (PMR)? The list goes on.

Claiming that FM is psychological is no defence either. When are we going to finally discard the outdated concept that psychological and physical illnesses are opposites? A huge body of research tells us that psychological and physical ill health move in tandem. What chronic illness does not affect us psychologically? Are newly diagnosed cancer patients not psychologically distraught? What about recent stroke victims? Does this make cancer and stroke psychological diseases? Of course not. The reality is that chronic physical illness begets chronic psychological distress, and vice versa. Numerous research studies have demonstrated alterations in physiologic function including immune response in those who are depressed(22-25). The dramatic increase in mortality in the year following the death of a spouse(26-28) is poignant evidence that psychological distress affects us physically. This is all part of the biopsychosocial understanding of illness, a concept that is far better supported by current research than the biomedical model so many of us were taught in medical school. Moreover, so-called *psychological disorders* are not without physiologic changes. Physiologic changes have been identified in and pharmacologic treatments justified for numerous psychiatric diagnoses including schizophrenia, major depression, bipolar disorder, obsessive-compulsive disorder, and attention deficit hyperactivity disorder, to name a few. As such, the distinction between physical and psychological illness becomes increasingly meaningless. The distinction between a physical symptom and a psychological one becomes more blurred. What is important is that all such patients are in distress, and that physicians can help (or hinder) if they so choose.

The callous disregard exhibited by some health care professionals (and others) for FM also is not defendable by arguing that the FM label is a distinctly poor one, although it is true that the FM label may be flawed. The tautologic (round-about) method by which FM was defined in 1990(29) (collecting a group of individuals believed to have FM and then looking for characteristics that distinguish them from those believed not to have FM) is the same scientific method that has been used to develop classification criteria for every other disorder (including SLE and RA) for which they exist. What other method might be employed in the absence of a gold standard confirmatory test? And what possible justification could there be to develop classification criteria for a disorder in which a gold standard confirmatory test already exists? The answer to both of these questions: there is none. The FM label, like those of SLE, RA, and many other disorders, may be tenuous. But that may just be the nature of the diagnostic labelling process itself.

The claim in medicine that we have 999 diseases is a myth. The truth is that we have 999 labels. Some of these labels, such as pneumococcal pneumonia or gout, work very well. FM, SLE, RA, PMR, and many other disorders that fall under the rheumatic disease umbrella are not well labelled. Nonetheless, these labels do serve many purposes. Certainly, there is very little discussion about discarding the SLE label, or the RA label, or the PMR label. Why must we discard the FM label? Despite arguments to the contrary, there is no evidence that the FM label is any more or less useful than those of SLE and RA.

The most oft-used argument has been that the FM label is harmful by creating illness behavior and disability, causing individuals to take on a 'sick role' and behave as if they are ill(19,28,30,31). But this argument is flawed at both ends. First, as has been shown repeatedly in controlled studies of FM patients versus controls, these people are ill. As stated earlier, the FM cohort differs physiologically from the normal population, in many instances in a physiologically predictable way. One would expect individuals reporting high levels of pain to have higher levels of neurotransmitter pain agonists in CSF, and FM patients do(15). One would expect individuals reporting non-restorative sleep to have electrophysiologic alterations in deep sleep, and FM patients do(9). In fact, as stated earlier, the number of alpha wave intrusions in Stage IV sleep is highly correlated with daytime symptoms(10). Hence, this cohort of patients with symptoms of illness and pathophysiologic changes consistent with illness, irrespective of their specificity, must be considered ill. Can you truly tell an individual complaining of feeling hot and having a core temperature of 40°C (104°F) that they are not ill because fever is not a specific finding?

And second, recently published research in a prospectively followed, representative community cohort of adults newly diagnosed with FM found that the FM label itself does not cause worsened future outcome(32). These individuals did not act more ill. They actually reported fewer symptoms over time. They did not use more health services. And the majority continued working. Hence, the FM label is flawed, admittedly. But it does not stand out in this regard. Numerous other diagnostic labels, such as SLE and RA, are equally flawed. Should they be discarded as well?

Perhaps the most volatile concept inducing venomous responses against FM is that of disability. This issue has not only medical, but also strong medicolegal implications. Some have argued that the only reason that FM exists is that an overly generous compensation system is in place that is ripe for the picking by individuals who claim to be too ill to work. (It takes no imagination at all to see how this anti-FM agenda might be pushed aggressively by those health care providers among us whose incomes come largely from performing independent medical evaluations for insurance companies.) However, evidence now exists to rebut even this contention.

The recently published study in which FM was found to be even more prevalent among Amish than non-Amish populations should serve as an antidote against such venom. Moreover, the finding of FM in the Amish should not be considered surprising. Previously published general representative (randomized) population studies have demonstrated FM to be more common in countries in which compensation availability might be expected to be less (for example, Pakistan(33), Poland(34), and South Africa(35)) than in countries in which compensation availability might be expected to be greater (Sweden(36), Denmark(37), and Finland(38)). Nonetheless, the venomous attacks continue(39,40). One author even insinuates that the motives of the Amish study investigators were purely political, and hence the results might somehow have been manipulated(41). And yet, the same author seems to take no exception to the endless armchair philosophizing of so many who have claimed, while making no attempt to gather any evidence to support their contentions, that FM is a compensation-driven illness.

Why? Why is FM unrelentingly held up to a level of scrutiny to which no other musculoskeletal disorder is held? Some authors, such as Ehrlich, Hadler, and A.S. Russell (42) (not to be confused with I.J. Russell, who has contributed greatly to our current understanding of FM through thoughtful, innovative research.) seem to have made a career out of writing opinion papers chastising FM, while publishing virtually no research at all to support any of their claims. Why? Why do those who belittle the concept of FM offer virtually nothing more of an argument than their own feeble versions of 'common sense', while repeatedly ignoring a huge and ever-growing body of evidence supporting its legitimacy?

I cannot answer for those who choose to utilize their positions of influence in this way. Nor can I answer for those who are much less verbal, but who choose to believe the armchair critics while exercising no effort to explore the research literature for themselves. But I believe that soon, the evidence supporting FM will become so insurmountable, so undeniable, that even the most violent FM-beaters will have to relent.

The answer is blowing in the wind and soon it will be felt. Technology ultimately will catch up with reality and will prove FM doubters wrong. We will be able to see and measure FM, in the clinical setting, just as relatively recent technological advances now allow us to measure hypothyroidism without goiter, and relapsing-remitting multiple sclerosis, two conditions whose pasts are not entirely unlike fibromyalgia's present. Hypothyroidism without goiter: how possibly could this have been diagnosed or conceptualized before we could test levels of thyroid function? These patients were just middle-aged, overweight, and lazy — or so it was thought. Relapsing-remitting multiple sclerosis: until the advent of magnetic resonance imaging and other technologies, these women were dismissed as being psychologically disturbed or malingerers, complaining of odd neurological symptoms like blindness and dizziness and drunken gait, yet appeared virtually neurologically intact on examination.

Let FM not be another tragic example of letting ill-informed, malicious logic derail conscientious, methodical attempts to gradually discover the truth. To quote Bob Dylan again:

"How many ears can one man have

before he can hear people cry?"

REFERENCES FOR

FIBROMYALGIA: THE ANSWER IS BLOWIN' IN THE WIND

1. Ochoa JL. Essence, investigation, and management of "neuropathic" pains: hopes from acknowledgement of chaos. Muscle Nerve 1993;16:997-1008. [MEDLINE]

2. Hart FD. Fibrositis (fibromyalgia): A common non-entity? Drugs 1988;35:320-7. [MEDLINE]

3. Gardner M. Fads and fallacies in the name of science. New York: Dover; 1957:86.

4. Hadler NM. The danger of the diagnostic process. In: Hadler NM, editor. Occupational musculoskeletal disorders. New York: Raven; 1993:16-33.

5. Block DR. Fibromyalgia and the rheumatisms. Common sense and sensibility. Rheum Dis Clin North Am 1993;19:61-78. [MEDLINE]

6. Anderson KN, Anderson LE, Glanze WD, editors. Mosby's medical, nursing and allied health dictionary. 4th ed. St. Louis: Mosby Year Book; 1994.

7. Dorland's medical dictionary. Philadelphia: W.B. Saunders; 1994.

8. Granges G, Littlejohn GO. A comparative study of clinical signs in fibromyalgia/fibrositis syndrome, healthy and exercising subjects. J Rheumatol 1993;20:344-51. [MEDLINE]

9. Moldofsky H. Sleep and fibrositis syndrome. Rheum Dis Clin North Am 1989;15:91-103. [MEDLINE]

10. Roizenblatt S, Moldofsky H, Benedito-Silva AA, Tufik S. Alpha sleep characteristics in fibromyalgia. Arthritis Rheum 2001;44:222-30. [MEDLINE]

11. McCain GA, Tilbe KS. Diurnal hormone variation in fibromyalgia syndrome. A comparison with rheumatoid arthritis. J Rheumatol 1989;16 Suppl 19:154-7.

12. Bennett RM, Clark SR, Campbell SM, Burckhardt CS. Low levels of somatomedin C in patients with the fibromyalgia syndrome. A possible link between sleep and muscle pain. Arthritis Rheum 1992;35:1113-6. [MEDLINE]

13. Yunus MB, Dailey JW, Aldag DC, Masi AT, Jobe PC. Plasma tryptophan and other amino acids in primary fibromyalgia: A controlled study. J Rheumatol 1992;19:90-4. [MEDLINE]

14. Russell IJ, Vaeroy H, Javors M, et al. Cerebrospinal fluid biogenic amine metabolites in fibromyalgia/fibrositis syndrome and rheumatoid arthritis. Arthritis Rheum 1992;35:550-6. [MEDLINE]

15. Vaeroy H, Helle R, Forre O, Kass E, Terenius L. Elevated CSF levels of substance P and high incidence of Raynaud's phenomenon in patients with fibromyalgia: new features for diagnosis. Pain 1988;32:21-6. [MEDLINE]

16. van West D, Maes M. Neuroendocrine and immune aspects of fibromyalgia. BioDrugs 2001;15:521-31. [MEDLINE]

17. Hau PP, Scudds RA, Harth M. An evaluation of mechanically induced neurogenic flare by infrared thermography in fibromyalgia. J Musculoskel Pain 1996;4:3-20.

18. Qiao Z, Vaeroy H, Morkrid L. Electrodermal and microcirculatory activity in patients with fibromyalgia during baseline, acoustic stimulation and cold pressor tests. J Rheumatol 1991;18:1383-9. [MEDLINE]

19. Martinez-Lavin M, Hermosillo AG, Mendoza C, et al. Orthostatic sympathetic derangement in subjects with fibromyalgia. J Rheumatol 1997;24:714-8. [MEDLINE]

20. Mountz JM, Bradley LA, Modell JG, et al. Fibromyalgia in women. Abnormalities of regional cerebral blood flow in the thalamus and the caudate nucleus are associated with low pain threshold levels. Arthritis Rheum 1995;38:926-38. [MEDLINE]

21. Bradley LA, Alberts KR, Alarcon GS, et al. Abnormal brain regional cerebral blood flow (rCBF) and cerebrospinal fluid (CSF) levels of substance P (SP) in patients and non-patients with fibromyalgia (FM) [abstract]. Arthritis Rheum 1996;39 Suppl:S212.

22. Irwin M, Clark C, Kennedy B, Christian Gillin J, Ziegler M. Nocturnal catecholamines and immune function in insomniacs, depressed patients, and control subjects. Brain Behav Immun 2003;17:365-72. [MEDLINE]

23. Jozuka H, Jozuka E, Takeuchi S, Nishikaze O. Comparison of immunological and endocrinological markers associated with major depression. J Int Med Res 2003;31:36-41. [MEDLINE]

24. Maddock C, Pariante CM. How does stress affect you? An overview of stress, immunity, depression and disease. Epidemiol Psychiatr Soc 2001;10:153-62. [MEDLINE]

25. Raison CL, Miller AH. The neuroimmunology of stress and depression. Semin Clin Neuropsychiatry 2001;6:277-94. [MEDLINE]

26. Tomassini C, Rosina A, Billari FC, Skytthe A, Christensen K. The effect of losing the twin and losing the partner on mortality. Twin Res 2002;5:210-7. [MEDLINE]

27. Martikainen P, Valkonen T. Mortality after the death of a spouse: rates and causes of death in a large Finnish cohort. I. Am J Public Health 1996;86:1087-93. [MEDLINE]
28. Smith KR, Zick CD. Risk of mortality following widowhood: age and sex differences by mode of death. Soc Biol 1996;43:59-71. [MEDLINE]

29. Wolfe F, Smythe HA, Yunus MB, et al. The American College of Rheumatology 1990 criteria for the classification of fibromyalgia. Report of the Multicenter Criteria Committee. Arthritis Rheum 1990;33:160-72. [MEDLINE]

30. Brena SR, Chapman SL: The 'learned pain syndrome': Decoding a patient's pain signals. Postgrad Med 1981;69:53-64. [MEDLINE]

31. Chapman SL, Brena SR. Learned helplessness and responses to nerve blocks in chronic low back patients. Pain 1982;14:355-64. [MEDLINE]

32. White KP, Nielson WR, Harth M, Speechley M, Ostbye T. Does the label 'fibromyalgia' alter health status and function? A prospective, within-group comparison [abstract]. Arthritis Rheum 2000;43 Suppl:S212.

33. Farooqi A, Gibson T. Prevalence of the major rheumatic disorders in the adult population of north Pakistan. Br J Rheumatol 1998;37:491-5. [MEDLINE]

34. The epidemiology of fibromyalgia: Workshop of the Standing Committee of Epidemiology, European League Against Rheumatism (EULAR), Bad Sackingen, 19-21 November 1992. Br J Rheumatol 1994;33:783-6.

35. Lyddell C, Meyers OL. The prevalence of fibromyalgia in a South African community [abstract]. Scand J Rheumatol 1992;Suppl 94:8.

36. Jacobsson L, Lindegard F, Manthorpe R. The commonest rheumatic complaints over a 6 weeks' duration in a twelve month period in a defined Swedish population. Scand J Rheumatol 1989;18:353-60. [MEDLINE]

37. Prescott E, Kjoller M, Jacobsen S, Bulow PM, Danneskiold-Samsoe B, Kamper-Jorgensen F. Fibromyalgia in the adult Danish population: I. A prevalence study. Scand J Rheumatol 1993; 22:233-7. [MEDLINE]

38. Makela M, Heliovaara M. Prevalence of primary fibromyalgia in the Finnish population. BMJ 1991;303:216-9. [MEDLINE]

39. Ehrlich GE. Pain is real; fibromyalgia isn't. J Rheumatol 2003;30:1666-7. [MEDLINE]

40. Hadler NM. "Fibromyalgia" and the medicalization of misery. J Rheumatol 2003;30:1668-70. [MEDLINE]

41. Wolfe F. Stop using the American College of Rheumatology criteria in the clinic. J Rheumatol 2003;30:1671-2. [MEDLINE]

42. Russell AS, Percy JS. Disabling fibromyalgia: appearance vs. reality [letter]. J Rheumatol 1994;21:1580.

SUPPLEMENTARY

MATERIALS

DR. WHITE'S BIBLIOGRAPHY

Publications

Editorials

1. **White KP**, Nielson W, Harth M: Psychological distress and health care seeking behaviour: caution warranted in interpreting data (Editorial). J Rheumatol 1999;26(2):244-6.

2. **White KP**: Fibromyalgia: The answer is blowin' in the wind. J Rheumatol, 2004;31: 636-9

Peer Reviewed Scientific Papers

1. **White KP**, McCain GA, Tunks E: The effects of changing the painful stimulus upon dolorimetry scores in patients with fibromyalgia. *J Musculoskeletal Pain* 1993;1(1):43-58.

2. **White KP**, Speechley M, Harth M, Ostbye T: Fibromyalgia in rheumatology practice: A survey of Canadian rheumatologists. *J Rheumatol* 1995;22(4):722-726.

3. **White KP**, Neilson WR: Cognitive behavioural treatment in fibromyalgia syndrome: A follow-up assessment. *J Rheumatol* 1995;22 (4):717-721.

4. **White KP**, Harth M: An analytical review of 24 controlled fibromyalgia (FMS) clinical trials. *Pain* 1996;64(2);211-219.

5. **White KP**, Harth M, Speechley M, Østbye T: Testing an instrument to screen for fibromyalgia syndrome in general population studies: The London Fibromyalgia Epidemiology Study Screening Questionnaire (LFESSQ). *J Rheumatol* 1998;26(4): 880-4.

6. **White KP**, Speechley M, Harth M, Østbye T: The London Fibromyalgia Epidemiology Study (LFES): Direct health care costs of fibromyalgia syndrome (FMS) in London, Ontario. *J Rheumatol* 1999;26:885-9.

7. **White KP**, Speechley M, Harth M, Østbye T: The London Fibromyalgia Epidemiology Study (LFES): Comparing self-reported function and work disability in 100 community cases of fibromyalgia syndrome versus controls in London, Ontario. *Arthritis Rheum* 1999;42(1):76-83.

8. **White KP**, Speechley M, Harth M, Østbye T: The London Fibromyalgia Epidemiology Study (LFES): The prevalence of fibromyalgia syndrome (FMS) in London, Ontario. *J Rheumatol* 1999;26:1570-6.

9. **White KP**, Speechley M, Harth M, Østbye T: The London Fibromyalgia Epidemiology Study (LFES): Comparing the demographic and clinical characteristics in 100 random community cases of fibromyalgia syndrome (FMS) versus controls. *J Rheumatol* 1999;26:1577-85.

10. **White KP**, Harth M, Speechley M, Østbye T: Fibromyalgia (FMS) tender points in FMS cases from the general population: Testing construct validity and reliability. J Rheumatol 2000;27(11):2677-82.

11. **White KP**, Speechley M, Harth M, Østbye T: Co-existence of chronic fatigue syndrome (CFS) with fibromyalgia syndrome (FMS) in the general population: A controlled study. Scand J Rheumatol 2000;29(1):44-51.

12. **White KP**, Østbye T, Harth M, Nielson W, Speechley M, Teasell R, Bourne R: Perspectives on post-traumatic fibromyalgia: A random survey of Canadian general practitioners, orthopedists, physiatrists and rheumatologists. J Rheumatol 2000;27:790-6.

13. **White KP**, Carette S, Harth M, Teasell RW. Trauma and fibromyalgia: Is there an association and what does it mean? Semin Arthritis Rheum 2000;29:200-16.

14. **White KP**, Nielson W, Harth M, Ostbye T, Speechley M: Chronic widespread musculoskeletal pain with or without fibromyalgia: Psychological distress in a representative community adult sample. J Rheumatol 2002 Mar;29(3):588-94

15. **White KP**, Harth M: Lumbar planus presenting as cauda equina syndrome in a patient with long-standing rheumatoid arthritis. J Rheumatol 2001;28:627-30.

16. **White KP**, Harth M, Speechley M, Ostbye T, Nielson W: A three year follow-up of a representative community sample of adults with chronic widespread pain, with or without fibromyalgia (FM). [in preparation]

17. Pankoff BA, Overend TJ, Lucy SD, **White KP:** Validity and responsiveness of the 6 minute walk test for people with fibromyalgia. J Rheumatol 2000; Nov;27(11): 2666-2670

18. Huisman AM, **White KP**, Algra A, Bell DA, Harth M, Vieth R, Jacobs JWG, Bijlsma WJ: Vitamin D in female systemic lupus erythematosis and fibromyalgia patients. *J Rheumatol* 2001; Nov;28(11):2535-9.

19. **White KP**, Harth M, Speechley M, Ostbye T: Does the label □*fibromyalgia*□ adversely affect clinical course and health service utilization? Arthritis Rheum 2002 Jun 15;47(3):260-5

20. Jones DA, Rollman B, **White KP**, Hill M, Brooks RI: Effect of catastrophizing on chronic pain outcomes. [Accepted in Journal of Pain]

21. Thomas AW, **White KP**, Drost DJ, Prato FS: A comparison of rheumatoid arthritis (RA) and fibromyalgia (FM) patients and healthy controls exposed to a pulsed (200uT) magnetic field: Effects on normal standing balance. *Neuroscience Letters* 200; Aug; 309(1): 17-20

22. Hill ML, Chiodo D, Bell DA, Harth M, le Riche N, Pope J, Thompson JL, **White KP**: Determining the need for allied health treatment services in the Rheumatology outpatient clinic: Patient-identified versus Rheumatologist-identified treatment needs. [in prep]

23. **White KP**, Thompson J: Fibromyalgia Syndrome (FMS) in an Amish Community of Southwestern Ontario (FACSO): A Controlled Study to determine disease and symptom prevalence. *J Rheum* 2003; 30(8):1835-40.

24. **White KP**: Developing and validating a clinical case definition for the fibromyalgia syndrome for use in clinical practice. *J Musculoskel Pain*, 2003;11:117-18.

Letters

1. **White KP**, Teasell R: Debating the use of SMRs {skeletal muscle relaxants}. *Can Fam Phys* 1994; 40(6):1089-1090.

2. **White KP**, Harth M: The Fibromyalgia Problem [letter]. *J Rheumatol* 1998;25(5):1022-1023.

3. **White KP**, Carette S, Harth M, Teasell RW. Trauma and fibromyalgia: Is there an association and what does it mean? Semin Arthritis Rheum 2000;29:200-16.

4. **White KP**, Harth M: To lump or to split. The importance of tender points. J Rheumatol, 2001;10:2362-2362

5. **White KP**, Harth M: Lumbar pannus in rheumatoid arthritis. J Rheumatol 2001 Mar;28(3):627-30

6. Harth M, **White KP**: Cauda Equina Syndrome or a Complication of Total Hip Arthroplasty. J of Rheum 2002; 39(1)

7. **White KP**, Harth M, Speechley M, Ostbye T: 'Fibromyalgia Label' – More pros than cons. Arthritis Care Res [submitted]

8. **White KP**, Harth M., Nielson W, Speechley M: Reply to the "Editor" Arthritis Rheum 2003 Feb 15;49(1):144-5

9. **White KP**: The Answer is Blowin' In the Wind: Response J. Rheumatol, 2004, 31(4):636-639

Book Reviews

1. **White, KP**. [Book Review] Osteoporosis: Diagnostic and Therapeutic Principles. J Rheum 1997;24(4):815.

2. **White KP**. [Book Review] Wounded Workers. The Politics of Musculoskeletal Injuries. Pain Res Manage 1999;4(1):11.

Chapters

1. **White KP**, Harth M. The occurrence and impact of generalized pain. Bailliere's Clinical Rheumatology. (Eds. Croft, Sillman) Harcourt Brace & Co., London, UK. 13:3. 01, 1999:379-89.

2. **White KP**, Harth M: Classification, Epidemiology and Natural History of Fibromyalgia. Current Science 2001; 1 *Curr Pain Headache Rep* 2001;Aug;5(4):320-9

3. **White KP**: The Epidemiology of Fibromyalgia. J Can Rheum Assoc,

2001;11:16-7.

4. **White KP, Harth M**: The differential diagnosis of Chronic Regional Pain. In Wallace DJ, Clauw DJ, eds, Fibromyalgia and Other Central Pain Syndromes. Lippincott, Williams & Wilkins, Philadelphia, 2005: 299-308

5. **White KP**: Developing and validating a clinical case definition for the fibromyalgia syndrome for use in clinical practice. The Fibromyalgia Syndrome. A Clinical Case Definition for Practitioners. Russell IJ, Editor. Haworth Medical Press, 2004:117-18.

6. **White KP**: Fibromyalgia and myofascial pain syndrome. Neurological Therapeutics: Principles and Practice, Volume 1. Noseworthy J, ed., 2006

Literature Reviews

1. Teasell R, **White KP**: Clinical approaches to low back pain. Part I. Epidemiology, diagnosis, and prevention. *Can Fam Phys* 1994;40: 481-486.

2. Teasell R, **White KP**: Clinical approaches to low back pain. Part II. Management, sequelae, and disability and compensation. *Can Fam Phys* 1994;40(3): 490-495.

3. **White KP**, Harth M, Teasell R: Work disability evaluation and the fibromyalgia syndrome. Semin Arthritis Rheum 2002 Oct;32(2):71-93

4. Masi A, **White KP**, Pilcher JJ: A person-centered approach to care, teaching and research in fibromyalgia syndrome: Justification from biopsychosocial perspectives in populations. *Semin Arthritis Rheum* 2002; 32(2): 71-93

5. **White KP**, Carette S, Harth M, Teasell RW: Trauma and fibromyalgia: Is there a connection and what does it mean? Semin Arthritis Rheum 2000;29:200-216(19;58)

GLOSSARY OF TERMS

Algesic: pain causing

Algometer: a spring-loaded device used to measure a patient's level of tenderness; see also, *dolorimeter*

American College of Rheumatology (ACR) Classification Criteria for FM: a list of criteria published by the ACR to aid in the classification of FM, primarily for research purposes; subsequently used by many to diagnose FM; require that the patient report at least three months of widespread pain (primarily in muscles) and have tenderness at no fewer than 11 of 18 body points that initially were identified in a large, multi-center clinical study of more than 260 FM patients versus a similar number of control patients without FM

Analgesic: pain relieving

Anti-nuclear antibodies: a blood test done to detect the presence of antibodies against cell nuclei; a screening test for systemic lupus erythematosus (lupus, SLE) and other diseases of the immune system

Arthritis: disease affecting the joints; numerous different types exist, including osteoarthritis, rheumatoid arthritis, systemic lupus, gout, etc.

Arthritis Impact Measurement Scale (AIMS): a questionnaire arthritis patients fill out that helps to assess how much their arthritis affects their daily activities and function

Autoimmune: a person's immune system attacks that person's own tissues; classic autoimmune diseases are lupus, rheumatoid arthritis and multiple sclerosis

Autonomic Nervous System: the part of the nervous system over which we have no to little voluntary control; it regulates such body functions as heart rate, blood pressure, pupil size, and sweating

Biomedical Model: the theoretical model that sees illness purely as the result of some anatomical or physiological abnormality; the traditional model of disease

Biopsychosocial model: the theoretical model of illness that sees illness as a complex interaction between a person's anatomy and/or physiology, emotional state, and social environment; a more recently developed and accepted model of disease

Black Lung Disease: lung disease caused by prolonged exposure to coal dust. In the 1950s, compensation for black lung disease was given to thousands with X-ray evidence of the condition, despite completely normal pulmonary (lung) function.

Hadler has made the case that the same mistake is being made with fibromyalgia and chronic pain.

Brain-Derived Neurotropic Peptide: a critical chemical that is involved in nerve survival and the plasticity of nerve synapses (see neuroplasticity).

Bursitis: a bursa is a fluid-filled sac that usually lies, like a pillow, between a muscle and some bony surface, so as to protect the muscle from wear and tear sustained while rubbing against the bone

Catecholamine-O-MethylTransferase (COMT): an enzyme important in the metabolism of neurotransmitters; some patients with fibromyalgia appear to have a genetic deficiency in COMT

Cervical spine: the neck

Chronic Fatigue Syndrome (CFS): also called myalgic encephalomyelitis; a condition similar to fibromyalgia, associated with severe fatigue, as well as numerous other symptoms that may include pain; as with fibromyalgia, is diagnosed using a list of criteria

Classification Criteria: a list comprised of patient symptoms and/or physical and/or laboratory signs that are used to define a given disease for which no definitive test exists

Control Points (for fibromyalgia): points on the body that some doctors use, in error, to tell if a fibromyalgia patient is faking or not; the concept of fibromyalgia control points has been scientifically disproven

Cortisol: an important hormone that has numerous bodily functions; levels are abnormal in fibromyalgia

De Quervain's tenosynovitis: a type of tendonitis of the wrist

Dolorimeter: a spring-loaded device used to measure a patient's level of tenderness; see also, *algometer.*

Dorsal Horn: part of the spinal cord that receives nerve input from peripheral sensory nerves

Dynorphin: a class of neurotransmitter that has opium-like actions

Epicondylitis (elbow): two painful conditions of the elbow; when it occurs on the outer elbow, known as *tennis elbow*; on the inner side, as *golfer's elbow*

Fascia: the thin lining that surrounds every muscle, it is richly innervated with sensory nerves

FC-42 (42-item fibromyalgia checklist): a questionnaire designed to assess the number, range and severity of symptoms in patients with fibromyalgia

Fibro fog: the mental fogginess that is so commonly reported by FM patients, primarily characterized by problems with short-term memory and concentration.

Fibrositis: an older name for fibromyalgia, now rarely used

Fibromyalgia Impact Questionnaire (FIQ): a questionnaire designed to assess the severity of several symptoms, overall severity, and impact upon daily activities in patients with fibromyalgia

Fibrous Tissue: body tissues like tendons, ligaments and fascia

Gold Standard Test: a definitive test; a positive result virtually confirms a given diagnosis

Greater Trochanteric Bursitis: a type of bursitis producing pain in the area of the outer hip and buttock (see bursitis)

Growth Hormone: a hormone that stimulates growth, but also aids in the repair of injured muscle; levels appear to be low in patients with fibromyalgia, especially at night when the repair of small muscle tears generally takes place

Health Assessment Questionnaire (HAQ): a questionnaire designed to assess the severity of several symptoms, overall severity, and impact upon daily activities in patients with arthritis

Hippocampus: an area of the brain that, among other things, is important in regulating sleep, pain perception, and some cognitive (thinking) processes; in fibromyalgia patients, blood flow to the hippocampus is less than normal

Hippocratic Oath: an oath by which doctors swear to practice medicine ethically, including the promise to 'do no harm'.

Hormone: a class of chemicals produced by the body to stimulate other, distant metabolic processes; for example, thyroid hormone stimulates such things as metabolic rate and heart rate; growth hormone stimulates growth in children and cell reproduction and regeneration

Hyperaemia: excessive blood flow

Hyperalgesia: increased sensitivity to pain; a lowered pain threshold

Incidence: the number of new cases of a given condition over a fixed period of time; most commonly, over one year.

Independent Medical Examination (IME): an examination performed by a physician or other healthcare giver, usually to assess for level of disability, for which the assessor is paid by some independent party (like the patient's insurance company or the patient's own lawyer)

Independent Medical Examiner: a physician or other healthcare giver who performs an IME.

Insulin-Like Growth Factor: a class of hormones that help to regulate the growth, development and regeneration of a broad variety of tissues, including nerves and muscles.

Irritable Bowel: also called *irritable bowel syndrome*; a condition classically associated with alternating constipation and non-bloody diarrhoea, often accompanied by crampy abdominal pain and other abdominal symptoms

Ischaemic Heart Disease: a condition in which there is chronically inadequate blood flow to the muscles of the heart

Ketanserine: a chemical that has a variety of functions, which include dilating (enlarging the diameter of) blood vessels, thereby reducing blood pressure and increasing blood flow.

Levator Scapula: a pair of muscles in the upper back that help to raise the shoulder blades (scapula)

Livido Reticularis: a skin condition in which the skin appears mottled (multi-coloured); classically associated with lupus, it is seen in many other conditions as well

Lumbosacral Spine: the lower spine

Lupus (systemic lupus erythematosus; SLE): an autoimmune condition in which a person's immune system attacks normal tissues; often associated with inflammatory arthritis and a variety of skin rashes, it can affect almost any organ system. Severe cases can be fatal

Met-enkephalin-Arg6-Phe7 (MEAP): one type of neurotransmitter

Motor Nerve: a nerve that stimulates muscle fibres to contract, often causing movement

Multiple Sclerosis: an autoimmune condition in which a person's immune system attacks the lining of nerves (called the myelin sheath) in the brain and spinal cord, resulting in loss of nerve function; it can be steadily progressive, relapsing and remitting, or some combination of these two courses

Musculoskeletal: pertaining to the muscles, bones and related tissues

Myofascial: pertaining to both muscle and fascia (see fascia)

Myofascial Pain Syndrome: a condition characterized by localized muscle pain and trigger points (see Trigger Point)

Nerve Growth Factor: a chemical (called a *neuropeptide*) that helps to stimulate and regulate nerve growth, development and regeneration

Nervous System: the brain, spinal cord and peripheral nerves

Neuron: a nerve cell

Neuroplasticity: permanent changes that occur within nerves, often as a result of an injury

Neurotransmitter: a class of chemicals that relay, amplify, and modulate signals between adjacent nerves; levels of several different neurotransmitters are abnormal in patients with fibromyalgia

N-methyl-aspartate: one type of neurotransmitter

N-methyl-D-aspartic Acid (NMDA) Receptor: it plays a role in what has been called pain *wind up*, whereby after an initial painful stimulus, subsequent equal stimuli are felt to be even more painful. These receptors are normally inactive; but, with repeated stimulation, they turn on. NMDA hyper-excitability and the ability to reduce that hyper-excitability using an NMDA receptor antagonist, called *ketanserin*, have been demonstrated in FM patients

Nociception: the nerve processes underlying the processing and encoding of noxious stimuli, like pain, extreme heat, extreme cold, etc.

Nociceptive Flexion Reflex: the extent to which a specific muscle in the leg withdraws in response to an electrical stimulus applied directly to the sural nerve of the leg

Opiates: a class of drugs that have pain-killing (analgesic) qualities; drugs like morphine, codeine and oxycodone are opiates; also called *narcotics*

Orthostatic Hypotension: a condition in which a person's blood pressure falls and heart rate increases excessively when they go from lying to sitting, and/or from sitting to standing; this often results in the person feeling light-headed, but some may faint; commonly seen in fibromyalgia patients

Osteoarthritis (OA): the most common form of arthritis, associated more with joint degeneration than inflammation

Pain Agonist: a type of neurotransmitter that increases one's perception of pain

Pain Antagonist: a type of neurotransmitter that decreases one's perception of pain

Pain-On, Pain-Off System: a system in which certain neurotransmitters are released first to increase someone's perception of pain, followed by other neurotransmitters to decrease it

Pathology: another word for disease

Pathophysiology: the underlying cause of disease, at a chemical/biological level

Phantom Limb: a limb that still is felt even after it has been amputated

Phantom Limb Pain: pain in a limb even after that limb (or part of the limb) has been amputated

Physiology: chemical/biological processes that occur in the body

Physiological: pertaining to chemical/biological processes that occur in the body

Placebo: a fake (inert or inactive) pill that is intended to look and taste exactly like the real active drug

Polymyalgia Rheumatica (PMR): a poorly-understood condition in which a person, usually elderly, gradually develops severe diffuse pain and stiffness that generally improves dramatically when they are given a steroid drug called prednisone; to date, why patients feel these symptoms is not known

Positive Predictive Value (PPV): the percentage of people correctly identified as having a given disease when a given test is positive

Post-Traumatic Fibromyalgia: fibromyalgia that starts soon after an injury, most commonly of the neck and/or back

Prevalence: the total number of ongoing cases of a given condition within a fixed population at one given time

Prolactin: a hormone; women with elevated prolactin levels are 15 times as likely to have fibromyalgia as women whose levels are normal

Prolylendopeptidase: an enzyme involved in the maturation and degradation of various pain-causing (algesic) neurotransmitters, like substance P; activity levels are reduced in FM patients

Prospective study: in a prospective study, all the data are collected AFTER the researchers have designed the study and decided what questions to ask. For example, a randomized clinical (drug) trial, where patients are assigned to either take an active drug or a placebo, is one type of prospective study

Psychosocial: pertaining to someone's psychological status and social environment

Pulmonary Hypertension: elevation of blood pressure within blood vessels feeding the lungs; a common component of diseases like scleroderma

Randomized clinical trial (RCT): this is the gold standard drug trial. In it, patients are randomly assigned to receive one treatment versus another (or versus a placebo), and then followed to see how they do. Once all the data are collected, the two groups are compared statistically

Raynaud's Phenomenon: a condition in which someone's hands turn bluish and abnormally cold in response to cold exposure; sometimes painful; it is seen more often than normal in persons with a variety of conditions, including lupus and fibromyalgia

Reactive Hyperaemia: excessive and prolonged redness and warmth of the skin following minor trauma like pinching the skin or pricking it with a pin; more common in individuals with versus those without fibromyalgia

Repetitive Strain Injury (RSI): chronic (long-standing) pain in a limb related to repetitive use; examples include carpal tunnel syndrome, tennis elbow (see epicondylitis), and rotator cuff tendonitis

Retrospective Study: this is a study where the researchers look at already-collected data; for example, they might review the medical charts of patients who already have been treated. This contrasts with a prospective study (see above).

Return-to-Work (RTW) Program: a program designed to return injured or chronically ill persons back into the workforce, generally by starting them off with a few hours per week and gradually increasing their hours; they are of unproven benefit in FM

Rheumatism: pain in muscles or other musculoskeletal tissue not caused by arthritis

Rheumatoid Arthritis (RA): the most common form of inflammatory arthritis

Rheumatoid Factor (RF): a test that is useful for diagnosing rheumatoid arthritis; however, used alone, it is neither sensitive nor specific

Rotator Cuff Tendonitis: a common form of tendonitis involving the shoulder

Sacroiliac Joints: a pair of joints just adjacent to and on either side of the lumbosacral spine in the low back

Saline: salt water

Scleroderma: an autoimmune condition associated with abnormally thickened skin and Raynaud's phenomenon; often accompanied by other problems

Sedimentation Rate (erythrocyte sedimentation rate, ESR): an extremely non-specific test that is positive in countless diseases

Sensitivity: a measure of how useful a given test, physical sign, or other diagnostic procedure is at identifying those with a given disease; high sensitivity means that almost everyone with the disease is positive for this test or sign; this contrasts with high specificity, where almost everyone with this test or sign has the disease.

Sensory Nerve: a nerve that brings sensory input (for example, cold, touch, or pain) back to the spinal cord and brain so it can be 'felt'.

Serotonin: a neurotransmitter and pain antagonist

Shingles: a sometimes excruciatingly painful condition that follows a specific viral rash

The **Snark:** a fictitious and ferocious creature created by the author Lewis Carol in his humorous poem called *The Hunting of the Snark*

Somatomedin C: another name for *insulin-like growth factor type I* (see insulin-like growth factor)

Specificity: a measure of how useful a given test, physical sign, or other diagnostic procedure is at identifying those with a given disease; high specificity means that almost every person with this test or sign has the disease; this contrasts with high sensitivity, which means that almost everyone with the disease is positive for this test or sign. *Example:* fever is very sensitive, but very non-specific for meningitis. Almost everyone with meningitis will have a fever; but very few people who have a fever have meningitis causing it.

Spinal Fluid (cerebrospinal fluid, CSF): fluid that surrounds the brain and spinal cord

Stage 4 Sleep: (also called *stage IV sleep*) the fourth of the five known stages of sleep; deep sleep that is associated with prominent delta wave electrical activity in the brain, and virtually no alpha wave activity; stage 4 sleep is markedly diminished in persons with fibromyalgia, and the degree of stage 4 loss is significantly correlated with the person's level of pain.

Substance P: a neurotransmitter and pain agonist; when released by nerves, it increases a person's perceived level of pain.

Symptom: a subjective sensation, usually of some disease state; for example, pain, nausea, dizziness, or fatigue

Tautology: circular reasoning

Tender Point: a point on the skin that hurts (is tender) when pushed upon

Tenderness: pain to touch or being pushed upon

Tendon: a fibrous tissue that connects muscle to bone

The Princess & the Pea: a famous story written by Hans Christian Anderson, in which the princess has trouble sleeping and is tender all over

Trapezius Muscle: a muscle that runs between the neck and shoulder

Trauma: injury

Trigeminal Neuralgia: a painful disorder involving the trigeminal nerve of the face; patients have facial pain

Trigger Point: a point on the skin that, when pushed upon, causes pain to radiate elsewhere (contrasts with a tender point, see above)

Tryptophan: a neurotransmitter and pain antagonist, related to serotonin

Urinary Frequency: having to urinate more often than normal, often associated with discomfort or pain, either in the lower abdomen or the urethra (the tube urine passes through when exiting the bladder)

Waddell's Signs: a series of physical tests initially designed to identify low back pain patients who were faking their pain; these tests have since been discredited, even by Dr. Waddell himself

Whiplash: a form of neck injury most commonly seen with rear-end car collisions, when the neck is rapidly and vigorously forced back and then forward.

LIST OF REFERENCED FIRST AUTHORS

Name	Reference(s)
Aaron, L. A.	(31)
Abeles, A. M.	(275)
Adigüzel, O.	(227)
Al-Allaf, A. W.	(403)
Alanoðlu, E.	(240)
Alarcon-Segovia, D.	(129)
Andren, L.	(285)
Anthony, K. K.	(159;164)
Arnett, F. C.	(201)
Arnold, L. M.	(266)
Assumpcao, A.	(132)
Baldursdóttir, S.	(155)
Baraniuk, J. N.	(282)
Bates, B.	(305)
Bayazit, Y. A.	(241)
Bazelmans, E.	(125)
Bengtsson, A.	(55)
Bennett, R. M.	(188;189;246;248;274;287)
Block, S. R.	(114)
Bohr, T. W.	(26;98)
Bradley, L. A.	(190;207;276)
Brena, S. R.	(324)
Brown, G. T.	(163)
Bruusgaard, D.	(377)
Buchwald, D.	(191)
Burckhardt, C. S.	(368;453)
Buskila, D.	(17;32;135;148;151;178;245;267)
Calabozo-Raluy,M	(363)
Calabro,J.J	(183)
Campbell,S.M	(14)
Cardiel,M.H	(130)
Carmona,L.	(126)
Chaimnuay,P	(142)
Chapman,S.L	(325)
Chobanian,A.V.	(205)
Clark,P.	(131)
Cohen,M.L	(200)
Cook,D.B.	(229;230)
Crofford,L.J.	(472)
Cruz, B. A.	(40)
Cuatrecasas,G.	(249)
Darmawan,J.	(143)

Qiao, Z.	(251)
Radloff, L.	(346)
Raspe, H.	(123)
Rau, C. L.	(303)
Reid, G. J.	(160;172)
Reilly, P. A.	(364)
Ribera, J. M.	(186)
Rice, J. R.	(101)
Robbins, J. M.	(326)
Robinson, R. L.	(445)
Roizenblatt, S.	(174;187)
Romano, T. J.	(33;36;37;182)
Rosenhall, U.	(242)
Rush, P. J.	(113)
Russell, I. J.	(74;193;211-213;473)
Saccomani, L.	(179)
Sack, J.	(115)
Salaffi, F.	(124)
Sandberg, M.	(254)
Sardini, S.	(175)
Schanberg, L. E.	(169)
Schmidt-Wilcke,T	(257-259)
Senecal, J. C.	(319)
Senna, E. R.	(133)
Sherry, D. D.	(165)
Siegal, D. M.	(170)
Simms, R. W.	(39;272;273;462)
Simons, D. G.	(96;97)
Sitges, C.	(233)
Small, E.	(162)
Smythe, H. A.	(12;29;108)
Spath, M.	(286)
Speilberger, C.	(347)
Staud, R.	(34;278;464;465;474;475)
Stevens, A.	(466)
Stockman, R.	(99)
Stratz, T.	(214)
Swaak, T.	(315)
Tan, E. M.	(202)
Tayag-Kier, C. E.	(166)
Thune, O.	(38)
Tisher, M.	(404)
Toda, K.	(144)
Topbas, M.	(134)
Travell, J. G.	(103)
Tunks, E.	(80;204)

Ulas, U. H.   (252)
Uveges, J. M.   (23)
Vaeroy, H.   (208)
Veerapen, K.   (141)
Vierck, C. J.   (304)
Walco, G. A.   (181)
Wallace, D. J.   (206)
Weigert, D. A.   (279)
White, K. P.
   (13;19;53;54;58;59;68;92;116;147;197;198;323;327;345;361;476)
Wig, G.   (234;235)
Wikner, J.   (289)
Williams, D. A.   (467)
Wolfe, F.
                (5;16;24;60-62;81;82;117;194-196;199;215;373)
Wood, P. B.   (468)
Wysenbeek, A. J.   (69)
Yoldas, T.   (469)
Yunus, M. B.   (2;3;25;184;216;269;470;481)
Zapata, A. L.   (149)

INDEX

B

C

D

E

I

J

N

Q

R

S

T

U

Reference List

(1) Gowers W. Lumbago: It's lessons and analogues. Br Med J 1904;1:117-21.

(2) Yunus MB, Masi AT, Aldag JC. A controlled study of primary fibromyalgia syndrome: clinical features and association with other functional syndromes. J Rheumatol 1989;16(suppl 19):62-71.

(3) Yunus M, Masi AT, Calabro JJ, et al. Primary fibromyalgia (fibrositis): clinical study of 50 patients with matched normal controls. Semin Arthritis Rheum 1981;11:151-71.

(4) Katz RS, Heard AR, Mills M, Leavitt F. The Prevalence and Clinical Impact of Reported Cognitive Difficulties (Fibrofog) in Patients With Rheumatic Disease With and Without Fibromyalgia. J Clin Rheumatol 2004;10(2):53-8.

(5) Wolfe F, Simons DG, Fiction J et al. The fibromyalgia and myofascial pain syndromes: a preliminary study of tender points and trigger points in persons with fibromyalgia, myofascial pain syndrome and no disease. J Rheumatol 1992;19:944-51.

(6) Kellgren JH. Observations on referred pain arising from muscle. Clin Sci 1938;3:175-90.

(7) Kellgren JH. On the distribution of pain arising from deep somatic structures with charts of segmental pain areas. Clin Sci 1939;4:35-46.

(8) Kellgren JH, McGowan AJ, Hughes ESR. On deep hyperalgesia and cold pain. Clin Sci 1944;7:13-27.

(9) Lewis T, Kellgren JH. Observations relating to referred pain, visceromotor reflexes and other associated phenomena. Clin Sci 1939;4:47-71.

(10) White KP, McCain GA, Tunks E. The effects of changing the painful stimulus upon dolorimetry scores in patients with fibromyalgia. J Musculoskeletal Pain 1993;1(1):43-58.

(11) Smythe HA, Buskila D, Urowitz S, Langevitz P. Control and "fibrositic" tenderness: comparison of two dolorimeters. J Rheumatol 1992;19(5):768-71.

(12) Smythe HA, Gladman A, Dagenais P et al. Relation between fibrositic and control site tenderness; effects of dolorimeter scale length and footplate size. J Rheumatol 1992;19(2):284-9.

(13) White KP, Speechley M, Harth M, Ostbye T. The London Fibromyalgia Epidemiology Study: The prevalence of fibromyalgia syndrome in London, Ontario. J Rheumatol 1999;19(7):1570-6.

(14) Campbell SM, Clark S, Tindall EA et al. Clinical characteristics of fibrositis. I. A "blinded" controlled study of symptoms and tender points. Arthritis Rheum 1983;26(7):817-24.

(15) Goldenberg DL. Fibromyalgia Syndrome: An Emerging but Controversial Condition. JAMA 1987;257(20):2782-7.

(16) Wolfe F, Hawley DJ, Cathey MA et al. Fibrositis: symptom frequency and criteria for diagnosis. An evaluation of 291 rheumatic disease patients and 58 normal individuals. J Rheumatol 1985;12(6):1159-63.

(17) Buskila D, Neumann L, Hershman E et al. Fibromyalgia syndrome in children - an outcome study. J Rheumatol 1995;22:525-8.

(18) Greenfield S, Fitzcharles M, Esdaile JM. Reactive fibromyalgia syndrome. Arthritis Rheum 1992;35(6):678-81.

(19) White KP, Carette S, Harth M, Teasell RW. Trauma and fibromyalgia: Is there a connection and what does it mean? Semin Arthritis Rheum 2000;29:200-16.

(20) Moldofsky H. Nonrestorative sleep and symptoms after a febrile illness in patients with fibrositis and chronic fatigue syndromes.
Moldofsky H. J Rheumatol Suppl 1989;19:150-3.

(21) Rea T, Russo J, Katon W et al. A prospective study of tender points and fibromyalgia during and after an acute viral infection. Arch Intern Med 1999;159(8):865-70.

(22) Scudds RA, Rollman GB, Harth M, et al. Pain perception and personality measures as discriminators in the classification of fibrositis. J Rheumatol 1987;14:563-9.

(23) Uveges JM, Parker JC, Smarr KL et al. Psychological symptoms in primary fibromyalgia syndrome: relationship to pain, life stress and sleep disturbance. Arthritis Rheum 1990;33:1279-83.

(24) Wolfe F, Cathey MA, Kleinheksel SM, et al. Psychological status in primary fibrositis and fibrositis associated with rheumatoid arthritis. J Rheumatol 1984;11:500-6.

(25) Yunus MB, Ahles TA, Aldag JC, et al. Relationship of clinical features with psychological status in primary fibromyalgia. Arthritis Rheum 1991;34:15-21.

(26) Bohr TW. Fibromyalgia syndrome and myofascial pain syndrome: do they exist? Neurol Clin 1995;13:365-84.

(27) Hart FD. Fibrositis (fibromyalgia): A common non-entity? Drugs 1988;35:320-7.

(28) Merskey H. Physical and psychological considerations in the classification of fibromyalgia. J Rheumatol 1989;15(suppl 19):72-9.

(29) Smythe HA. Problems with the MMPI. J Rheumatol 1994;11:417-8.

(30) Mufson M, Regestein QR. The spectrum of fibromyalgia disorders. Arthritis Rheum 1993;36:647-50.

(31) Aaron LA, Bradley LA, Alarcon GS et al. Psychiatric diagnoses in patients with fibromyalgia are related to health care-seeking behaviour rather than to illness. Arthritis Rheum 1996;39(3):436-45.

(32) Buskila D, Neumann L, Odes LR et al. The prevalence of musculoskeletal pain and fibromyalgia in patients hospitalized on internal medicine wards. Semin Arthritis Rheum 2001;30(6):411-7.

(33) Romano TJ. Coexistence of fibromyalgia syndrome (FS) and systemic lupus erythematosis (SLE). Scand J Rheumatol 1992;suppl 94:12.

(34) Staud R. Are patients with systemic lupus erythematosus at increased risk for fibromyalgia? Curr Rheumatol Rep 2006;8(6):430-5.

(35) Middleton GD, McFarlin JE, Lipsky PE. The prevalence and clinical impact of fibromyalgia in systemic lupus erythematosus. Arthritis Rheum 1994;37(8):1181-8.

(36) Romano TJ. Incidence of fibromyalgia syndrome (FS) in rheumatoid arthritis (RA) patients in a general rheumatology practice. Scand J Rheumatol 1992;94(Suppl):11.

(37) Romano TJ. Presence of fibromyalgia syndrome (FS) in osteoarthritis (OA) patients. Scand J Rheumatol 1992;suppl 94:11.

(38) Thune O. The prevalence of fibromyalgia among patients with psoriasis. Acta Derm Venereol 2005;85(1):33-7.

(39) Simms RW, Zerbini CAF, Ferrante N et al. Fibromyalgia Syndrome in patients infected with Human Immunodeficiency Virus. Amer J Med 1992;92:368-74.

(40) Cruz BA, Catalan-Soares B, Proietti F. Higher prevalence of fibromyalgia in patients infected with human T cell lymphotropic virus type I. J Rheumatol 2006;33(11):2300-3.

(41) Buskila D, Fefer P, Harman-Boehm I et al. Assessment of nonarticular tenderness and prevalence of fibromyalgia in hyperprolactinemic women. J Rheumatol 1993;20(12):2112-5.

(42) Jurell KC, Zanetos MA, Orsinelli A et al. Fibromyalgia: A Study of Thyroid Function and Symptoms. J Musculoskel Pain 1996;4(3):49-60.

(43) Fiona D, Esdaile JM, Kimoff JR, Fitzcharles M. Musculoskeletal complaints and fibromyalgia in patients attending a respiratory sleep disorders clinic. J Rheumatol 1996;23(9):1612-6.

(44) May KP, West SG, Baker MR, Everett DW. Sleep apnea in males with the fibromyalgia syndrome. Am J Med 1993;94:505-8.

(45) Sendur OF, Gurer G, Bozbas GT. The frequency of hypermobility and its relationship with clinical findings of fibromyalgia patients. Clin Rheumatol 2007;26(4):485-7.

(46) Ofluoglu D, Gunduz OH, Kul-Panza E, Guven Z. Hypermobility in women with fibromyalgia syndrome. Clin Rheumatol 2006;25(3):291-3.

(47) Acasuso-Diaz M, Collantes-Estevez E. Joint hypermobility in patients with fibromyalgia syndrome. Arthritis Care Res 1998;11(1):39-42.

(48) Hudson N, Starr MR, Esdaile JM, Fitzcharles M. Diagnostic associations with hypermobility in rheumatology patients. Br J Rheumatol 1995;34(12):1157-61.

(49) Gedalia A, Press J, Klein M, Buskila D. Joint hypermobility and fibromyalgia in schoolchildren. Ann Rheum Dis 1993;52(7):494-6.

(50) Granges G, Zilko P, Littlejohn GO. Fibromyalgia syndrome: Assessment of the severity of the condition two years after diagnosis. J Rheumatol 1994;21:523-9.

(51) Felson DT, Goldenberg DL. The natural history of fibromyalgia. Arthritis Rheum 1986;29:1522-6.

(52) Felson DT. Epidemiology of the Rheumatic Diseases. In: Koopman WJ, editor. Arthritis and Allied Conditions: A Textbook of Rheumatology, 14th Edition, Volume 1.Philadephia, PA: Lippincott, Williams & Wilkins; 2001. p. 3-38.

(53) White KP, Speechley M, Harth M, Ostbye T. Remission Rate in Fibromyalgia Syndrome (FMS). (Presented in poster format at the XII Pan-American Congress of Rheumatology, June 21-25, 1998, Montreal, Quebec.). 1998.

(54) White KP, Harth M. Classification, epidemiology, and natural history of fibromyalgia. Curr Pain Headache Rep 2001;5(4):320-9.

(55) Bengtsson A, Backman E. Long-term follow up of fibromyalgia patients. Scand J Rheumatol 1992;S94:98.

(56) Forseth KO, Førre O, Gran JT. A 5.5 year prospective study of self-reported musculoskeletal pain and of fibromyalgia in a female population: significance and natural history. Clin Rheumatol 1999;18(2):114-21.

(57) Kennedy M, Felson DT. A prospective long-term study of fibromyalgia syndrome. Arthritis Rheum 1996;39(4):682-5.

(58) White KP, Harth M, Teasell RW. Work disability evaluation and the fibromyalgia syndrome. Semin Arthritis Rheum 1995;24(6):371-81.

(59) White KP. Fibromyalgia: the answer is blowin' in the wind. J Rheumatol 2004;31(4):636-9.

(60) Wolfe F, Potter J. Fibromyalgia and work disability: Is fibromyalgia a disabling disorder? Rheum Dis Clin North Am 1996;22(2):369-91.

(61) Wolfe F, the Vancouver Fibromyalgia Consensus Group. The fibromyalgia syndrome: A consensus report on fibromyalgia and disability. J Rheumatol 1996;23:534-9.

(62) Wolfe F. The fibromyalgia problem. [Editorial]. J Rheumatol 1997;24:1247-9.

(63) Holmes GP, Kaplan JE, Gantz NM et al. Chronic fatigue syndrome: a working case definition. Ann Intern Med 1988;108(3):387-9.

(64) Reeves WC, Wagner D, Nisenbaum R et al. Chronic fatigue syndrome--a clinically empirical approach to its definition and study. BMC Med 2005 Dec 15;3:19 2005;15(3):19(1)-19(9).

(65) Fukuda K, Straus SE, Hickie I et al. The chronic fatigue syndrome: a comprehensive approach to its definition and study. International Chronic Fatigue Syndrome Study Group. Ann Intern Med 1994;121:953-9.

(66) Goldenberg DL. Fibromyalgia and chronic fatigue syndrome. J Musculoskeletal Pain 1994;2(3):51-5.

(67) Demitrack MA. Chronic fatigue syndrome and fibromyalgia. Dilemmas in diagnosis and clinical management. Psychiatr Clin North Am 1998;21(3):671-92.

(68) White KP, Speechley M, Harth M, Ostbye T. Co-existence of chronic fatigue syndrome with fibromyalgia syndrome in the general population. A controlled study. Scand J Rheumatol 2000;29(1):44-51.

(69) Wysenbeek AJ, Shapira Y, Leibovici L. Primary fibromyalgia and the chronic fatigue syndrome. Rheumatol Int 1991;10(6):227-9.

(70) Hudson JI, Goldenberg DL, Pope HG et al. Comorbidity of fibromyalgia with medical and psychiatric disorders. Amer J Med 1992;92(4):363-7.

(71) Goldenberg DL, Simms RW, Gieger A, Komaroff AL. High frequency of fibromyalgia in patients with chronic fatigue seen in primary care practice. Arthritis Rheum 1990;33:381-7.

(72) Goldenberg DL. Fibromyalgia and its relation to chronic fatigue syndrome, viral illness and immune abnormalities. J Rheumatol 1989;19(Suppl):91-3.

(73) Evengard B, Nilsson CG, Lindh G et al. Chronic fatigue syndrome differs from fibromyalgia. No evidence for elevated substance P levels in cerebrospinal fluid of patients with chronic fatigue syndrome. Pain 1998;78(2):153-5.

(74) Russell IJ, Orr MD, Litman B et al. Elevated cerebrospinal fluid levels of substance P in patients with the fibromyalgia syndrome. Arthritis Rheum 1994;37:1593-601.

(75) Lombardi VC, Ruscetti FW, Das Gupta J et al. Detection of an infectious retrovirus, XMRV, in blood cells of patients with chronic fatigue syndrome. Science 2009;326(5952):585-9.

(76) Hadler NM. Fibromyalgia: La maladie est morte. Vive le malade. J Rheumatol (editorial) 1977;24:1250-1.

(77) Hadler NM. "Fibromyalgia" and the medicalization of misery. J Rheumatol 2003;30(8):1668-70.

(78) Granges G, Littlejohn GO. Pressure pain threshold in pain-free subjects, in patients with chronic regional pain syndromes, and in patients with fibromyalgia syndrome. Arthritis Rheum 1993;36(5):642-6.

(79) Khostantine I, Tunks ER, Goldsmith CH, Ennis J. Fibromyalgia: can one distinguish it from simulation? An observer-blind controlled study. J Rheumatol 2000;27(11):2671-6.

(80) Tunks E, Crook J, Norman G, Kalaher S. Tender points in fibromyalgia. Pain 1988;34(1):11-9.

(81) Wolfe F, Smythe HA, Yunus M et al. The American College of Rheumatology 1990 criteria for the classification of fibromyalgia: report of the multicenter criteria committee. Arthritis Rheum 1990;33:160-72.

(82) Wolfe F. What use are fibromyalgia control points? Wolfe F. J Rheumatol 1998;25(3):546-50.

(83) Wolfe F, Clauw DJ, Fitzcharles M et al. The American College of Rheumatology Preliminary Diagnostic Criteria for Fibromyalgia and Measurement of Symptom Severity. Arthritis Care Res 2010;62(5):600-10.

(84) Harth M, Nielson WR. The fibromyalgia tender points: use them or lose them? A brief review of the controversy. J Rheumatol 2007;34(5):914-22.

(85) Ochoa JL. Essence, Investigation, and Management of "Neuropathic" Pains: Hopes from Acknowledgement of Chaos. Muscle Nerve 1993;16:977-1008.

(86) Gardner M. Fads and fallacies in the name of science. New York, NY: Dover; 1957.

(87) The Oxford Desk Dictionary: American Edition. New York, NY: Oxford University Press; 1995.

(88) Syndrome. Wikipedia 2010 March 24;Available from: URL: http://en.wikipedia.org/wiki/Syndrome

(89) Dorland's Illustrated Medical Dictionary, 31st edition. Philadelphia, PA: W.B. Saunders Company; 2007.

(90) Symptom. Wikipedia 2010;Available from: URL: http://en.wikipedia.org/wiki/Symptom

(91) Hadler NM. The danger of the diagnostic process. Occupational Musculoskeletal Disorders. New York, USA: Raven; 1993. p. 16-33.

(92) White KP, Nielson WR, Harth M et al. Does the label "fibromyalgia" alter health status, function, and health service utilization? A prospective, within-group comparison in a community cohort of adults with chronic widespread pain. Arthritis Rheum 2002;47(3):260-5.

(93) Job. The Book of Job. The Oxford Holy Bible. London: Oxford University Press; 1970. p. 726.

(94)   Spink R. Hans Andersen's Fairy Tales [translated]. New York, NY: E.P. Dutton & Co., Inc.; 1958.

(95)   Inanici F, Yunus M. History of fibromyalgia: past to present. Curr Pain Headache Rep 2004;8:369-78.

(96)   Simons DG. Muscle pain syndromes - Part I. Amer J Phys Med 1975;54:289-311.

(97)   Simons DG. Muscle pain syndromes - Part II. Amer J Phys Med 1976;55:15-42.

(98)   Bohr T. Problems with myofascial pain syndrome and fibromyalgia syndrome. Neurology 1996;46:593-7.

(99)   Stockman R. The causes, pathology and treatment of chronic rheumatism. Edinb Med J 1904;15:107-16.

(100) Kraft GH, Johnson EW, LaBan MM. The fibrositis syndrome. Arch Phys Med Rehab 1968;3:155-62.

(101) Rice JR. "Fibrositis ' syndrome. Med Clin N Amer 1986;70(2):455-68.

(102) Kellgren JH. Deep pain sensibility. Lancet 1949;1(6562):943-9.

(103) Travell JG, Simons DG. Myofascial pain and dysfunction. The trigger point manual. Baltimore, MD: Williams and Wilkins; 1983.

(104) Moldofsky H, Scarisbrick P, England R, Smythe HA. Musculoskeletal symptoms and non-REM sleep disturbance in patients with 'fibrositis syndrome' and healthy subjects. Psychosom Med 1975;37:341-51.

(105) Moldofsky H, Scarisbrick P. Induction of neurasthenic musculoskeletal pain by selective sleep stage deprivation. Psychosom Med 1976;38:35-44.

(106) Moldofsky H, Scarisbrick P. Induction of neurasthenic musculoskeletal pain syndrome by selective sleep stage deprivation. Psychosom Med 1976;38(1):35-44.

(107) Moldofsky H, Lue FA. The relationship of alpha and delta EEG frequencies to pain and mood in 'fibrositis' patients treated with chlorpromazine and L-tryptophan. Electroencephalogr Clin Neurophysiol 1980;50((1-2)):71-80.

(108) Smythe HA, Moldofsky H. Two contributions to an understanding of the 'fibrositis' syndrome. Bull Rheum Dis 1977;28(1):928-31.

(109) Hughes G, Martinez C, Myon E et al. The impact of a diagnosis of fibromyalgia on health care resource use by primary care patients in the UK: an observational study based on clinical practice. Arthritis Rheum 2006;54(1):117-83.

(110) Katz RS, Wolfe F, Michaud K. Fibromyalgia diagnosis: a comparison of clinical, survey, and American College of Rheumatology criteria. Arthritis Rheum 2006;54(1):169-76.

(111)   Ehrlich GE. Pain is real; fibromyalgia isn't. J Rheumatol 2003;30:1666-7.

(112)   Hadler NM. Social Security. The process of pensioning the invalid. In: Hadler NM, editor. Occupational Musculoskeletal Disorders. New York, USA: Raven Press; 1993. p. 227-48.

(113)   Rush PJ, Ameis A. The diseases which have no clothes: fibromyalgia and myofascial syndrome. Hippocrates Lantern 1997;3(3):1-5.

(114)   Block SR. Fibromyalgia and the rheumatisms. Common sense and sensibility. Rheum Dis Clin North Am 1993;19(1):61-78.

(115)   Sack J, Payne V. Alberta judge denies existence of fibromyalgia. Ont Med Rev 1995;67-73.

(116)   White KP, Harth M. The occurrence and impact of generalized pain. Baillieres Best Pract Res Clin Rheumatol 1999;13(3):379-89.

(117)   Wolfe F, Ross K, Anderson J et al. The prevalence and characteristics of fibromyalgia in the general population. Arthritis Rheum 1995;38:19-28 1995;38(1):19-28.

(118)   The Epidemiology of fibromyalgia: Workshop of the Standing Committee on Epidemiology European League Against Rheumatism (EULAR), Bad Sackingen, 19-21 November 1992. Brit J Rheumatol 1994;33:783-6.

(119)   Jacobsson L, Lindgarde F, Manthorpe R. The commonest rheumatic complaints of over 6 weeks' duration in a twelve month period in a defined Swedish population. Scand J Rheumatol 1989;18:361-8.

(120)   Lindell L, Bergman S, Petersson IF et al. Prevalence of fibromyalgia and chronic widespread pain. Scand J Prim Health Care 2000;18(3):149-53.

(121)   Makela M, Heliovaara M. Prevalence of primary fibromyalgia in the Finnish population. BMJ 1991;303:216-9.

(122)   Prescott E, Kjoller M, Jacobsen S et al. Fibromyalgia in the adult Danish population: I. A prevalence study. Scand J Rheumatol 1993;22:233-7.

(123)   Raspe H, Baumgartner CH. The epidemiology of fibromyalgia syndrome (FM) in a German town. Scand J Rheumatol 1992;94(Suppl):8.

(124)   Salaffi F, De Angelis R, Grassi W et al. Prevalence of musculoskeletal conditions in an Italian population sample: results of a regional community-based study. I. The MAPPING study. Clin Exp Rheumatol 2005;23(6):819-28.

(125)   Bazelmans E, Vercoulen JH, Galama JM et al. [Prevalence of chronic fatigue syndrome and primary fibromyalgia syndrome in The Netherlands] [Article in Dutch]. Ned Tijdschr Geneeskd 1997;141(31):1520-3.

(126)   Carmona L, Ballina J, Gabriel R et al. The burden of musculoskeletal diseases in the general population of Spain: results from a national survey. Ann Rheum Dis 2001;60(11):1040-5.

(127) Mas AJ, Carmona L, Valverde M et al. Prevalence and impact of fibromyalgia on function and quality of life in individuals from the general population: results from a nationwide study in Spain. Clin Exp Rheumatol 2008;26(4):519-26.

(128) Forseth KO, Gran JT. The prevalence of fibromyalgia among women aged 20-49 years in Arendal, Norway. Scand J Rheumatol 1992;21(2):74-8.

(129) Alarcon-Segovia D, Ramos-Niembro F, Gonzales-Amaro RF. One Thousand Private Rheumatology Patients in Mexico City. Arthritis Rheum 1983;26:688-9 [letter].

(130) Cardiel MH, Rojas-Serrano J. Community based study to estimate prevalence, burden of illness and help seeking behavior in rheumatic diseases in Mexico City. A COPCORD study. Clin Exp Rheumatol 2002;20(5):617-24.

(131) Clark P, Burgos-Vargas R, Medina-Palma C et al. Prevalence of fibromyalgia in children: a clinical study of Mexican children. J Rheumatol 1998;25(10):2009-14.

(132) Assumpcao A, Cavalcante AB, Capela CE et al. Prevalence of fibromyalgia in a low socioeconomic status population. BMC Musculoskelet Disord 2009;10:64-70.

(133) Senna ER, De Barros AL, Silva EO et al. Prevalence of rheumatic diseases in Brazil: a study using the COPCORD approach. J Rheumatol 2004;31(3):594-7.

(134) Topbas M, Cakirbay H, Gulec H et al. The prevalence of fibromyalgia in women aged 20-64 in Turkey. Scand J Rheumatol 2005;34(2):140-4.

(135) Buskila D, Neumann L, Vaisberg G et al. Increased rates of fibromyalgia following cervical spine injury. A controlled study of 161 cases of traumatic injury. Arthritis Rheum 1997;40(3):446-52.

(136) Peleg R, Ablin JN, Peleg A et al. Characteristics of fibromyalgia in Muslim Bedouin women in a primary care clinic. Semin Arthritis Rheum 2008;37(6):398-402.

(137) Kaki AM. Pain clinic experience in a teaching hospital in Western, Saudi Arabia. Relationship of patient's age and gender to various types of pain. Saudi Med J 2006;27(12):1882-6.

(138) Lyddell C, Meyers OL. The prevalence of fibromyalgia in a South African community. Scand J Rheumatol 1992;94(Suppl):8.

(139) Farooqi A, Gibson T. Prevalence of the major rheumatic disorders in the adult population of north Pakistan. Br J Rheumatol 1998;37:491-5.

(140) Haq SA, Darmawan J, Islam MN et al. Prevalence of rheumatic diseases and associated outcomes in rural and urban communities in Bangladesh: a COPCORD study. J Rheumatol 2005;32(2):348-53.

(141) Veerapen K, Wigley RD, Valkenburg H. Musculoskeletal pain in Malaysia: a COPCORD survey. J Rheumatol 2007;34(1):207-13.

(142) Chaimnuay P, Darmawan J, Muirden KD, Assawatanabodee P. Epidemiology of Rheumatic
       Disease in Rural Thailand: A WHO-ILAR COPCORD study. Community Oriented Programme
       for the Control of Rheumatic Disease. J Rheumatol 2010;25:1382-7.

(143) Darmawan J, Valkenburg HA, Muirden KD, Wigley RD. Epidemiology of Rheumatic Diseases
       in Rural and Urban Populations in Indonesia: A World Health Organization International
       League Against Rheumatism COPCORD Study, Stage 1, Phase 2. Annals Rheumatic Dis
       1992;51:525-8.

(144) Toda K. The prevalence of fibromyalgia in Japanese workers. Scand J Rheumatol
       2007;36(2):140-4.

(145) Zeng QY, Chen R, Darmawan J et al. Rheumatic diseases in China. Arthritis Res Ther
       2008;10(1):R17.

(146) Felson DT. Comparing the prevalence of rheumatic diseases in China with the rest of the
       world. Arthritis Res Ther 2008;10(1):106.

(147) White KP, Thompson J. Fibromyalgia syndrome in an Amish community: a controlled study
       to determine disease and symptom prevalence. J Rheumatol 2003;30(8):1835-40.

(148) Buskila D, Neumann L, Hazanov I, Carmi R. Familial aggregation in the fibromyalgia
       syndrome. Semin Arthritis Rheum 1996;26(3):605-11.

(149) Zapata AL, Moraes AJ, Leone C et al. Pain and musculoskeletal pain syndromes related to
       computer and video game use in adolescents. Eur J Pediatr 2006;165(6):408-14.

(150) Zijdenbos AP, Forghani R, Evans AC. Automatic "pipeline" analysis of 3-D MRI data for
       clinical trials: application to multiple sclerosis. IEEE Trans Med Imaging 2002;21:1280-91.

(151) Buskila D. Pediatric fibromyalgia. Rheum Dis Clin North Am 2009;35(2):253-61.

(152) Kashikar-Zuck S, Lynch AM, Slater S et al. Family factors, emotional functioning, and
       functional impairment in juvenile fibromyalgia syndrome. Arthritis Rheum
       2008;59(10):1392-8.

(153) Eccleston C. Children with chronic widespread pain: hunting the snark. Pain
       2008;138(3):477-8.

(154) Kashikar-Zuck S, Parkins IS, Graham TB et al. Anxiety, mood, and behavioral disorders among
       pediatric patients with juvenile fibromyalgia syndrome. Clin J Pain 2008;24(7):620-6.

(155) Baldursdóttir S. [Juvenile primary fibromyalgia syndrome--review] [Article in Icelandic].
       Laeknabladid 2008;94(6):463-72.

(156) Michels H, Gerhold K, Hafner R et al. [Juvenile fibromyalgia syndrome] [Article in German].
       Schmerz 2008;22(3):339-48.

(157)   Eraso RM, Bradford NJ, Fontenot CN et al. Fibromyalgia syndrome in young children: onset at age 10 years and younger. Clin Exp Rheumatol 2007;25(4):639-44.

(158)   Kashikar-Zuck S, Lynch AM, Graham TB et al. Social functioning and peer relationships of adolescents with juvenile fibromyalgia syndrome. Arthritis Rheum 2007;57(3):474-80.

(159)   Anthony KK, Schanberg LE. Pediatric pain syndromes and management of pain in children and adolescents with rheumatic disease. Pediatr Clin North Am 2005;52(2):611-39.

(160)   Reid GJ, McGrath PJ, Lang BA. Parent-child interactions among children with juvenile fibromyalgia, arthritis, and healthy controls. Pain 2005;113((1-2)201):210.

(161)   Kashikar-Zuck S, Vaught MH, Goldschneider KR et al. Depression, coping, and functional disability in juvenile primary fibromyalgia syndrome. J Pain 2002;3(5):412-9.

(162)   Small E. Chronic musculoskeletal pain in young athletes. Pediatr Clin North Am 2002;49(3):655-62.

(163)   Brown GT, Delisle R, Gagnon N, Sauve AE. Juvenile fibromyalgia syndrome: proposed management using a cognitive-behavioral approach. Phys Occup Ther Pediatr 2001;21(1):19-36.

(164)   Anthony KK, Schanberg LE. Juvenile primary fibromyalgia syndrome. Curr Rheumatol Rep 2001;3(2):165-71.

(165)   Sherry DD. Pain syndromes in children. Curr Rheumatol Rep 2000;2(4):337-42.

(166)   Tayag-Kier CE, Keenan GF, Scalzi LV et al. Sleep and periodic limb movement in sleep in juvenile fibromyalgia. Pediatrics 2000;106(5):E70.

(167)   Gedalia A, Garcia CO, Molina JF et al. Fibromyalgia syndrome: experience in a pediatric rheumatology clinic. Clin Exp Rheumatol 2000;18(3):415-9.

(168)   Mikkelsson M. One year outcome of preadolescents with fibromyalgia. J Rheumatol 1999;26(3):674-82.

(169)   Schanberg LE, Keefe FJ, Lefebre JC et al. Social context of pain in children with Juvenile Primary Fibromyalgia Syndrome: parental pain history and family environment. Clin J Pain 1998;14(2):107-15.

(170)   Siegel DM, Janeway D, Baum J. Fibromyalgia syndrome in children and adolescents: clinical features at presentation and status at follow-up. Pediatrics 1998;101((3 Pt 1)):377-82.

(171)   Mikkelsson M, Salminen JJ, Kautiainen H. Non-specific musculoskeletal pain in preadolescents. Prevalence and 1-year persistence. Pain 1997;73(1):29-35.

(172)   Reid GJ, Lang BA, McGrath PJ. Primary juvenile fibromyalgia: psychological adjustment, family functioning, coping, and functional disability. Arthritis Rheum 1997;40(4):752-60.

(173) Kashikar-Zuck S, Graham TB, Huenefeld MD, Powers SW. A review of biobehavioral research in juvenile primary fibromyalgia syndrome. Arthritis Care Res 2000;13(6):388-97.

(174) Roizenblatt S, Tufik S, Goldenberg J et al. Juvenile fibromyalgia: clinical and polysomnographic aspects. J Rheumatol 1997;24(3):579-85.

(175) Sardini S, Ghirardini M, Betelemme L et al. [Epidemiological study of a primary fibromyalgia in pediatric age] [Article in Italian]. Minerva Pediatr 1996;48(12):543-50.

(176) Gare BA. Epidemiology of rheumatic disease in children. Curr Opin Rheumatol 1996;8(5):449-54.

(177) Gedalia A, Press J, Klein M, Buskila D. Joint hypermobility and fibromyalgia in schoolchildren. Ann Rheum Dis 1993;52(7):494-6.

(178) Buskila D, Press J, Gedalia A et al. Assessment of nonarticular tenderness and prevalence of fibromyalgia in children. J Rheumatol 1993;20(2):368-70.

(179) Saccomani L, Vigliarolo MA, Sbolgi P et al. [Juvenile fibromyalgia syndrome: 2 clinical cases] [Article in Italian]. Pediatr Med Chir 1993;15(1):99-101.

(180) Malleson PN, al-Matar M, Petty RE. Idiopathic musculoskeletal pain syndromes in children. J Rheumatol 1992;19(11):1786-9.

(181) Walco GA, Ilowite NT. Cognitive-behavioral intervention for juvenile primary fibromyalgia syndrome. J Rheumatol 1992;19(10):1617-9.

(182) Romano TJ. Fibromyalgia in children; diagnosis and treatment. W V Med J 1991;87(3):112-4.

(183) Calabro JJ. Fibromyalgia (fibrositis) in children. Am J Med 1986;81(3A):57-9.

(184) Yunus MB, Masi AT. Juvenile primary fibromyalgia syndrome. A clinical study of thirty-three patients and matched normal controls. Arthritis Rheum 1985;28(2):138-45.

(185) Kasapcopur O, Tengirsek M, Ercan G et al. Hypermobility and fibromyalgia frequency in childhood familial Mediterranean fever. Clin Exp Rheumatol 2004;22((4 Suppl 34)):79.

(186) Ribera JM, Oriol A. Acute lymphoblastic leukemia in adolescents and young adults. Hematol Oncol Clin North Am 2009;23(5):1033-42.

(187) Roizenblatt S, Moldofsky H, Benedito-Silva AA, Tufik S. Alpha sleep characteristics in fibromyalgia. Arthritis Rheum 2001;44(1):222-30.

(188) Bennett RM. Fibromyalgia: the commonest cause of widespread pain. Compr Ther 1995;21(6):269-75.

(189) Bennett RM, Jones J, Turk DC et al. An internet survey of 2,596 people with fibromyalgia. BMC Musculoskelet Disord 2007;8:27.

(190)   Bradley LA, McKendree-Smith NL, Alarcón GS. Pain complaints in patients with fibromyalgia versus chronic fatigue syndrome.
Bradley LA, McKendree-Smith NL, Alarcón GS. Curr Rev Pain 2000;4(2):148-57.

(191)   Buchwald D. Fibromyalgia and chronic fatigue syndrome: similarities and differences. Rheum Dis Clin North Am 1996;22(2):219-43.

(192)   McCain GA. Diagnosis and treatment of fibromyalgia. In: Teasell R SA, editor. Cervical Flexion-Extension/Whiplash Injuries. Toronto: 1993. p. 423-41.

(193)   Russell IJ. Is fibromyalgia a distinct clinical entity? The clinical investigator's evidence. Baillieres Best Pract Res Clin Rheumatol 1999;13(3):445-54.

(194)   Wolfe F, Cathey MA. Prevalence of primary and secondary fibrositis. J Rheumatol 1983;10:965-8.

(195)   Wolfe F. The Clinical Syndrome of Fibrositis. Amer J Med 1986;81(3A):7-14.

(196)   Wolfe F. Fibromyalgia: The clinical syndrome. Rheum Dis Clin North Am 1989;15(1):1-18.

(197)   White KP, Speechley M, Harth M, Ostbye T. The London Fibromyalgia epidemiology study: comparing the demographic and clinical characteristics in 100 random community cases of fibromyalgia versus controls. J Rheumatol 1999;26(7):1577-85.

(198)   White KP, Speechley M, Harth M, Ostbye T. Comparing self-reported function and work disability in 100 community cases of fibromyalgia syndrome versus controls in London, Ontario: the London Fibromyalgia Epidemiology Study. Arthritis Rheum 1999;42(1):76-83.

(199)   Wolfe F, Ross K, Andersen J, Russell IJ. Aspects of fibromyalgia in the general population: sex, pain threshold, and fibromyalgia symptoms. J Rheumatol 1995;22(1):151-6.

(200)   Cohen ML, Quintner JL. Fibromyalgia syndrome, a problem of tautology. Lancet 1993;342(8876):906-9.

(201)   Arnett FC, Edworthy SM, Bloch DA, et al. The American Rheumatism Association 1987 revised criteria for the classification of rheumatoid arthritis. Arthritis Rheum 1988;31:315-24.

(202)   Tan EM, Cohen AS, Fries JF et al. The 1982 revised criteria for the classification of systemic lupus erythematosus. Arthritis Rheum 1082;25(11):1271-7.

(203)   Dasgupta B, Salvarani C, Schirmer M et al. Developing classification criteria for polymyalgia rheumatica: comparison of views from an expert panel and wider survey. J Rheumatol 2008;35(2):270-7.

(204)   Tunks E, McCain GA, Hart LE et al. The reliability of examination for tenderness in patients with myofascial pain, chronic fibromyalgia and controls. J Rheumatol 1995;22:944-52.

(205)   Chobanian AV, Bakris GL, Black HR, et al. The Seventh Report of the Joint National Committee on Prevention, Detection, Evaluation, and Treatment of High Blood Pressure: the JNC 7 report. JAMA 2003;289(19):2560-72.

(206)   Wallace DJ. Systemic Lupus Erythematosis, Rheumatology and Medical Literature: Current Trends. J Rheum 1985;12:913-5.

(207)   Bradley LA, Alberts KR, Alarcon GS, et al. Abnormal brain regional cerebral blood flow (rCBF) and cerebrospinal fluid (CSF) levels of substance P (SP) in patients and non-patients with fibromyalgia (FM). Arthritis Rheum 1996;39(9 (suppl)):S212.

(208)   Vaeroy H, Helle R, Forre O et al. Elevated CSF levels of substance P and high incidence of Raynaud phenomenon in patients with fibromyalgia: new features for diagnosis. Pain 1988;32:21-6.

(209)   Russell IJ, Larson AA. Neurophysiopathogenesis of fibromyalgia syndrome: a unified hypothesis. Rheum Dis Clin N Am 2009;35(2):421-35.

(210)   Moldofsky H, Warsh JJ. Plasma tryptophan and musculoskeletal pain in non-articular rheumatism ("fibrositis syndrome"). Pain 1978;5(1):65-71.

(211)   Russell IJ, Mickalek JE, Vipraio GA et al. Serum amino acids in fibrositis/fibromyalgia syndrome. J Rheumatol Suppl 1989;19:158-63.

(212)   Russell IJ. Neurohormonal aspects of fibromyalgia syndrome. Rheum Dis Clin North Am 1989;15(1):149-68.

(213)   Russell IJ, Vaeroy H, Javors M, Nyberg F. Cerebrospinal fluid biogenic amine metabolites in fibromyalgia/fibrositis syndrome and rheumatoid arthritis. Arthritis Rheum 1992;35(5):550-6.

(214)   Stratz T, Samborski W, Hrycaj P et al. [Serotonin concentration in serum of patients with generalized tendomyopathy (fibromyalgia) and chronic polyarthritis] [Article in German]. Med Klin (Munich) 1993;88(8):458-62.

(215)   Wolfe F, Russell IJ, Vipraio GA et al. Serotonin levels, pain threshold, and fibromyalgia symptoms in the general population. J Rheumatol 1997;24(3):555-9.

(216)   Yunus MB, Dailey JW, Aldag JC et al. Plasma tryptophan and other amino acids in primary fibromyalgia: a controlled study. J Rheumatol 1992;19(1):90-4.

(217)   Neeck G. Neuroendocrine and hormonal perturbations and relations to the serotonergic system in fibromyalgia patients. Scand J Rheumatol Suppl 2000;113:8-12.

(218)   De Stefano R, Selvi E, Villanova M et al. Image analysis quantification of substance P immunoreactivity in the trapezius muscle of patients with fibromyalgia and myofascial pain syndrome. J Rheumatol 2000;27(12):2906-10.

(219) Elvin A, Siosteen AK, Nilsson A, Kosek E. Decreased muscle blood flow in fibromyalgia patients during standardised muscle exercise: a contrast media enhanced colour Doppler study. Eur J Pain 2006;10(2):137-44.

(220) McIver KL, Evans C, Kraus RM et al. NO-mediated alterations in skeletal muscle nutritive blood flow and lactate metabolism in fibromyalgia. Pain 2006;120((1-2)):161-9.

(221) Guedj E, Cammilleri S, Colavolpe C et al. Predictive value of brain perfusion SPECT for ketamine response in hyperalgesic fibromyalgia. Eur J Nucl Med Mol Imaging 2007 Mar 13 [Epub ahead of print] 2007.

(222) Guedj E, Taieb D, Cammilleri S et al. (99m)Tc-ECD brain perfusion SPECT in hyperalgesic fibromyalgia. Eur J Nucl Med Mol Imaging 2007;34(1):130-4.

(223) Guedj E, Cammilleri S, Niboyet J et al. Clinical correlate of brain SPECT perfusion abnormalities in fibromyalgia. J Nucl Med 2008;49(11):1798-803.

(224) Kwiatek R, Barnden L, Tedman R et al. Regional cerebral blood flow in fibromyalgia: single-photon-emission computed tomography evidence of reduction in the pontine tegmentum and thalami. Arthritis Rheum 2000;43(12):2823-33.

(225) Mountz JM, Bradley LA, Modell JG, et al. Fibromyalgia in women. Abnormalities of regional cerebral blood flow in the thalamus and the caudate nucleus are associated with low pain threshold levels. Arthritis Rheum 1995;38(7):926-38.

(226) Mountz JM, Bradley LA, Alarcón GS. Abnormal functional activity of the central nervous system in fibromyalgia syndrome. Am J Med Sci 1998;315(6):385-96.

(227) Adigüzel O, Kaptanoglu E, Turgut B, Nacitarhan V. The possible effect of clinical recovery on regional cerebral blood flow deficits in fibromyalgia: a prospective study with semiquantitative SPECT. South Med J 2007;97(7):651-5.

(228) Gur A, Karakoc M, Erdogan S et al. Regional cerebral blood flow and cytokines in young females with fibromyalgia. Clin Exp Rheumatol 2002;20(6):753-60.

(229) Cook DB, Lange G, Ciccone DS et al. Functional imaging of pain in patients with primary fibromyalgia. J Rheumatol 2004;31(2):364-78.

(230) Cook DB, Stegner AJ, McLoughlin MJ. Imaging pain of fibromyalgia. Curr Pain Headache Rep 2007;11(3):190-200.

(231) Montoya P, Sitges C, García-Herrera M et al. Abnormal affective modulation of somatosensory brain processing among patients with fibromyalgia. Psychosom Med 2005;67(6):957-63.

(232) Montoya P, Sitges C, García-Herrera M et al. Reduced brain habituation to somatosensory stimulation in patients with fibromyalgia. Arthritis Rheum 2006;54(6):1995-2003.

(233) Sitges C, García-Herrera M, Pericás M et al. Abnormal brain processing of affective and sensory pain descriptors in chronic pain patients. J Affect Disord 2007 Apr 13 [Epub ahead of print] 2007.

(234) Wik G, Fischer H, Bragée B et al. Retrosplenial cortical activation in the fibromyalgia syndrome. Neuroreport 2003;14(4):619-21.

(235) Wik G, Fischer H, Finer B et al. Retrospenial cortical deactivation during painful stimulation of fibromyalgic patients. Int J Neurosci 2006;116(1):1-8.

(236) Gracely RH, Petzke F, Wolf JM, Clauw DJ. Functional magnetic resonance imaging evidence of augmented pain processing in fibromyalgia. Arthritis Rheum 2002;46(5):1333-43.

(237) Lekander M, Fredrikson M, Wik G. Neuroimmune relations in patients with fibromyalgia: a positron emission tomography study. Neurosci Lett 2000;282(3):193-6.

(238) Moldofsky H. Sleep and pain. Sleep Med Rev 2001;5(5):385-96.

(239) Moldofsky H. The significance of dysfunctions of the sleeping/waking brain to the pathogenesis and treatment of fibromyalgia syndrome. Rheum Dis Clin North Am 2009;35(2):275-83.

(240) Alanoðlu E, Ulaº UH, Ozdað F et al. Auditory event-related brain potentials in fibromyalgia syndrome. Rheumatol Int 2005;25(5):345-9.

(241) Bayazit YA, Gürsoy S, Ozer E et al. Neurotologic manifestations of the fibromyalgia syndrome. J Neurol Sci 2002;196(1-2):77-80.

(242) Rosenhall U, Johansson G, Orndahl G. Otoneurologic and audiologic findings in fibromyalgia. Scand J Rehabil Med 1996;28(4):225-32.

(243) McCain GA, Tilbe KS. Diurnal hormone variation in fibromyalgia syndrome. A comparison with rheumatoid arthritis. J Rheumatol 1989;16(suppl 19):154-7.

(244) McLean SA, Williams DA, Harris RE et al. Momentary relationship between cortisol secretion and symptoms in patients with fibromyalgia. Arthritis Rheum 2005;52(11):3660-9.

(245) Buskila D, Fefer P, Harman-Boehm I et al. Assessment of nonarticular tenderness and prevalence of fibromyalgia in hyperprolactinemic women. J Rheumatol 1993;20(12):2112-5.

(246) Bennett RM, Clark SR, Campbell SM, Burckhardt CS. Low levels of somatomedin C in patients with the fibromyalgia syndrome. A possible link between sleep and muscle pain. Arthritis Rheum 1992;35(10):1113-6.

(247) Leal-Cerro A, Povedano J, Astorga R et al. The growth hormone (GH)-releasing hormone-GH-insulin-like growth factor-1 axis in patients with fibromyalgia syndrome. J Clin Endocrinol Metab 1999;84(9):3378-81.

(248) Bennett RM, Cook DM, Clark SR et al. Hypothalamic-pituitary-insulin-like growth factor-I axis dysfunction in patients with fibromyalgia. J Rheumatol 1997;24(7):1384-9.

(249) Cuatrecasas G, Riudavets C, Guell MA, Nadal A. Growth hormone as concomitant treatment in severe fibromyalgia associated with low IGF-1 serum levels. A pilot study. BMC Musculoskelet Disord 2007;8:119.

(250) Hau PP, Scudds RA, Harth M. An evaluation of mechanically induced neurogenic flare by infrared thermography in fibromyalgia. J Musculoskel Pain 1997;4(3):3-20.

(251) Qiao Z, Vaeroy H, Morkrid L. Electrodermal and microcirculatory activity in patients with fibromyalgia during baseline, acoustic stimulation and cold pressor tests. J Rheumatol 1991;18(9):1383-9.

(252) Ulas UH, Unlu E, Hamamcioglu K et al. Dysautonomia in fibromyalgia syndrome: sympathetic skin responses and RR interval analysis. Rheumatol Int 2006;26(5):383-7.

(253) Martinez-Lavin M, Hermosillo AG, Mendoza C, et al. Orthostatic sympathetic derangement in subjects with fibromyalgia. J Rheumatol 1997;24(4):714-8.

(254) Sandberg M, Lindberg LG, Gerdle B. Peripheral effects of needle stimulation (acupuncture) on skin and muscle blood flow in fibromyalgia. Eur J Pain 2004;8(2):163-71.

(255) Granges G, Littlejohn GO. A comparative study of clinical signs in fibromyalgia/fibrositis syndrome, healthy and exercising subjects. J Rheumatol 1993;20(2):344-51.

(256) Laske C, Stransky E, Eschweiler GW et al. Increased BDNF serum concentration in fibromyalgia with or without depression or antidepressants. J Psychiatr Res 2007;41(7):600-5.

(257) Schmidt-Wilcke T, Luerding R, Weigand T et al. Striatal grey matter increase in patients suffering from fibromyalgia - A voxel-based morphometry study. Pain Jun 21 [Epub ahead of print] 2007.

(258) Schmidt-Wilcke T, Leinisch E, Straube A et al. Gray matter decrease in patients with chronic tension type headache. Neurology 2005;65:1483-6.

(259) Schmidt-Wilcke T, Leinisch E, Ganssbauer S et al. Affective components and intensity of pain correlate with structural differences in gray matter in chronic back pain patients. Pain 2006;125:89-97.

(260) Park JH, Phothimat P, Oates CT et al. Use of P-31 magnetic resonance spectroscopy to detect metabolic abnormalities in muscles of patients with fibromyalgia. Arthritis Rheum 1998;41:406-13.

(261) Ge HY. Prevalence of Myofascial Trigger Points in Fibromyalgia: The Overlap of Two Common Problems.
Ge HY. Curr Pain Headache Rep 2010 Jul 6 [Epub ahead of print] 2010.

(262) Ge HY, Wang Y, Danneskiold-Samsoe B et al. The predetermined sites of examination for tender points in fibromyalgia syndrome are frequently associated with myofascial trigger points. J Pain 2010;11(7):644-51.

(263) Ge HY, Nie H, Madeleine P et al. Contribution of the local and referred pain from active myofascial trigger points in fibromyalgia syndrome. Pain 2009;147((1-3)):233-40.

(264) Morf S, Amann-Vesti B, Forster A et al. Microcirculation abnormalities in patients with fibromyalgia - measured by capillary microscopy and laser fluxmetry. Arthritis Res Ther 2005;7(2):R209-R216.

(265) Frodin T, Bengtsson A, Skogh M. Nail fold capillaroscopy findings in patients with primary fibromyalgia. Clin Rheumatol 1988;7:384-8.

(266) Arnold LM, Hudson JI, Hess EV et al. Family study of fibromyalgia. Arthritis Rheum 2004;50(3):944-52.

(267) Buskila D, Neumann L. Fibromyalgia syndrome (FM) and nonarticular tenderness in relatives of patients with FM. J Rheumatol 1997;24(5):941-4.

(268) Harris RE, Clauw DJ. How do we know that the pain in fibromyalgia is "real"? Curr Pain Headache Rep 2006;10(6):403-7.

(269) Yunus MB, Khan MA, Rawlings KK et al. Genetic linkage analysis of multicase families with fibromyalgia syndrome. J Rheumatol 1999;26:408-12.

(270) Buskila D, Neumann L. Genetics of fibromyalgia. Curr Pain Headache Rep 2005;9(5):313-5.

(271) Denko CW, Malemud CJ. Serum growth hormone and insulin but not insulin-like growth factor-1 levels are elevated in patients with fibromyalgia syndrome. Rheumatol Int 2005;25(2):146-51.

(272) Simms RW. Is there muscle pathology in fibromyalgia syndrome? Rheum Dis Clin North Am 1996;22(2):245-66.

(273) Simms RW. Fibromyalgia is not a muscular disease. Am J Med Sci 1998;315:346-50.

(274) Bennett RM. Physical fitness and muscle metabolism in the fibromyalgia syndrome: An overview. J Rheumatol 1989;16(Suppl 19):28-9.

(275) Abeles AM, Pillinger MH, Solitar BM, Abeles M. Narrative review: the pathophysiology of fibromyalgia. Ann Intern Med 2007;146(10):726-34.

(276) Bradley LA, McKendree-Smith NL, Alberts KR et al. Use of neuroimaging to understand abnormal pain sensitivity in fibromyalgia. Curr Rheumatol Rep 2000;2(2):141-8.

(277) Johansson G, Risberg J, Rosenhall U et al. Cerebral dysfunction in fibromyalgia: evidence from regional cerebral blood flow measurements, otoneurological tests and cerebrospinal fluid analysis. Acta Psychiatr Scand 1995;91(2):86-94.

(278) Staud R, Rodriguez ME. Mechanisms of disease: pain in fibromyalgia syndrome. Nat Clin Pract Rheumatol 2006;2(2):90-8.

(279) Weigert DA, Bradley LA, Blalock JE, Alarcon GS. Current concepts in the pathophysiology of abnormal pain perception in fibromyalgia. Am J Med Sci 1998;315:405-12.

(280) Zimmerman M. Pathophysiological mechanisms of fibromyalgia. Clinical Journal of Pain 1991;7((suppl 7)):S8-S15.

(281) Melzack R, Wall PD. The challenge of pain. 2nd ed. London, England: Penguin Books; 1988.

(282) Baraniuk JN, Whalen G, Cunningham J, Clauw DJ. Cerebrospinal fluid levels of opioid peptides in fibromyalgia and chronic low back pain. BMC Musculoskelet Disord 2004;5:48.

(283) Graven-Nielson T, Aspegren Kendall S, Henriksson KG et al. Ketamine reduces muscle pain, temporal summation, and referred pain in fibromyalgia patients. Pain 2000;85(3):483-91.

(284) Sorensen J, Graven-Nielson T, Henriksson KG et al. Hyperexcitability in fibromyalgia. J Rheumatol 1998;25(1):152-5.

(285) Andren L, Svensson A, Dahlof B et al. Ketanserin in hypertension. Early clinical evaluation and dose finding study of a new 5-HT2 receptor antagonist. Acta Med Scand 1983;214(2):125-30.

(286) Späth M. Current experience with 5-HT3 receptor antagonists in fibromyalgia. Rheum Dis Clin North Am 2002;28(2):319-28.

(287) Bennett RM, Clark SC, Walczyk J. A randomized, double-blind, placebo-controlled study of growth hormone in the treatment of fibromyalgia. Am J Med 2010;104:227-31.

(288) Davidson JR, Moldofsky H, Lue FA. Growth hormone and cortisol secretion in relation to sleep and wakefulness. J Psychiatry Neurosci 1991;16:96-102.

(289) Wikner J, Hirsch U, Wetterberg L, Rojdmark S. Fibromyalgia--a syndrome associated with decreased nocturnal melatonin secretion. Clin Endocrinol (Oxf) 1998;49(2):179-83.

(290) Emad Y, Ragab Y, Zeinhom F et al. Hippocampus dysfunction may explain symptoms of fibromyalgia syndrome. A study with single-voxel magnetic resonance spectroscopy. J Rheumatol 2008;35(7):1371-7.

(291) Tang JS, Qu CL, Huo FQ. The thalamic nucleus submedius and ventrolateral orbital cortex are involved in nociceptive modulation: a novel pain modulation pathway. Prog Neurobiol 2009;89(4):383-9.

(292) Frese A, Husstedt IW, Ringelstein EB, Evers S. Pharmacologic treatment of central post-stroke pain. Clin J Pain 2006;22(3):252-60.

(293) Nicholson BD. Evaluation and treatment of central pain syndromes. Neurology 2004;62((5 Suppl 2)):S30-S36.

(294)   Katayama Y, Yamamoto T, Kobayashi K et al. Deep brain and motor cortex stimulation for post-stroke movement disorders and post-stroke pain. Acta Neurochir Suppl 2003;87:121-3.

(295)   Herrero MT, Barcia C, Navarro JM. Functional anatomy of thalamus and basal ganglia. Childs Nerv Syst 2002;18(8):386-404.

(296)   Segatore M. Understanding central post-stroke pain. J Neurosci Nurs 1996;28(1):28-35.

(297)   Davis RA, Stokes JW. Neurosurgical attempts to relieve thalamic pain. Surg Gynecol Obstet 1966;123(2):371-84.

(298)   San Pedro EC, Mountz JM, Mountz JD et al. Familial painful restless legs syndrome correlates with pain dependent variation of blood flow to the caudate, thalamus, and anterior cingulate gyrus. J Rheumatol 1998;25(11):2270-5.

(299)   Katz J, Melzack R. Pain "memories" in phantom limbs: review and clinical observations. Pain 1990;43:319-436.

(300)   Sumpton JE, Moulin DE. Fibromyalgia: presentation and management with a focus on pharmacological treatment. Pain Res Manag 2008;13(6):477-83.

(301)   Marcus DA. Current trends in fibromyalgia research. Expert Opin Pharmacother 2003;4(10):1687-95.

(302)   Crofford LJ, Clauw DJ. Fibromyalgia: where are we a decade after the American College of Rheumatology classification criteria were developed? Arthritis Rheum 2002;46(5):1136-8.

(303)   Rau CL, Russell IJ. Is fibromyalgia a distinct clinical syndrome? Curr Rev Pain 2000;4(4):287-94.

(304)   Vierck CJ. Mechanisms underlying development of spatially distributed chronic pain (fibromyalgia). Pain 2006;124(3):242-63.

(305)   Bates B. A Guide to Physical Examination, 2nd Edition. U.S.A.: J. P. Lippincott Company; 1979.

(306)   Skljarevski V, Ramadan NM. The nociceptive flexion reflex in humans - review article. Pain 2002;96:3-8.

(307)   Sandrini G, Serrao M, Rossi P et al. The lower limb flexion reflex in humans. Prog Neurobiol 2005;77:353-95.

(308)   Willer JC. Comparative study of perceived pain and nociceptive flexion reflex in man. Pain 1977;3:69-80.

(309)   Desmeules JA, Cedraschi C, Rapiti E et al. Neurophysiologic evidence for a central sensitization in patients with fibromyalgia. Arthritis Rheum 2003;48:1420-9.

(310) Banic B, Peetersen-Felix S, Andersen OK et al. Evidence for spinal cord hypersensitivity in chronic pain after whiplash injury and in fibromyalgia. Pain 2004;107:7-15.

(311) Froriep R. On the therapeutic application of electro-magnetism in the treatment of rheumatic and paralytic affections. Translated by Lawrence RM. London, U.K.: Henry Renshaw; 1850.

(312) Hochberg MC. Updating the American College of Rheumatology revised criteria for the classification of systemic lupus erythematosis. Arthritis Rheum 1997;40:1725.

(313) Causes of Malar Rash. WrongDiagnosis 10 A.D. March 12;Available from: URL: http://www.wrongdiagnosis.com/symptoms/malar_rash/causes.htm

(314) Edworthy SM, Zatarain E, McShane DJ, Bloch DA. Analysis of the 1982 ARA lupus criteria data set by recursive partitioning methodology: new insights into the relative merit of individual criteria. J Rheumatol 1988;15(10):1493-8.

(315) Swaak T, Smeenk R. Detection of anti-dsDNA as a diagnostic tool: a prospective study in 441 non-systemic lupus erythematosus patients with anti-dsDNA antibody (anti-dsDNA). Ann Rheum Dis 1985;44(4):245-51.

(316) Migliorini P, Baldini C, Rocchi V, Bombardieri S. Anti-Sm and anti-RNP antibodies. Autoimmunity 2005;38(1):47-54.

(317) Petri M, Magder L. Classification criteria for systemic lupus erythematosus: a review. Lupus 2004;13(11):829-37.

(318) Petri M. Review of classification criteria for systemic lupus erythematosus. Rheum Dis Clin North Am 2005;31(2):245-54.

(319) Senécal JC. Lupus: The Disease with a Thousand Faces. Lupus Canada 2009;Available from: URL: http://www.lupuscanada.org/english/living/1000faces.html

(320) Landrigan PJ. What causes autism? Exploring the environmental contribution. Curr Opin Pediatr 2010 Jan 16 [Epub ahead of print] 2010.

(321) The History of MS. AMSEL 2010; Available from: URL: http://www.historyofms.org/

(322) Majithia V, Geraci SA. Rheumatoid arthritis: diagnosis and management. Am J Med 2007;120(11):936-9.

(323) White KP. An Epidemiologic Study of Fibromyalgia in a Representative Community Sample: The London Fibromyalgia Epidemiology Study (LFES) - Doctoral Thesis University of Western Ontario; 1998.

(324) Brena SR, Chapman SL. The 'learned pain syndrome': Decoding a patient's pain signals. Postgrad Med 1981;69:53-64.

(325)   Chapman SL, Brena SR. Learned helplessness and responses to nerve blocks in chronic low
        back patients. Pain 1982;14:355-64.

(326)   Robbins JM, Kirmayer LS. Illness, worry and disability in fibromyalgia syndrome. Intl J Psych
        Med 1990;20:49-63.

(327)   White KP, Harth M, Speechley M, Ostbye T. Testing an instrument to screen for fibromyalgia
        syndrome in general population studies: the London Fibromyalgia Epidemiology Study
        Screening Questionnaire. J Rheumatol 1999;26(4):880-4.

(328)   Hadler NM. A critical appraisal of the fibrositis concept. Am J Med 1981;81(Suppl 3A):26-30.

(329)   Winfield JB. Fibromyalgia: what's next? [editorial]. Arthritis Care Res 1997;24:1247-9.

(330)   Wolfe F. Fibromyalgia. Rheum Dis Clin North Am 1990;16:681-98.

(331)   Hudson JI, Pope HGJr. Fibromyalgia and psychopathology: is fibromyalgia a form of
        "affective spectrum disorder"? J Rheumatol Suppl 1989;19:15-22.

(332)   Hudson JI, Pope HGJr. The relationship between fibromyalgia and major depressive disorder.
        Rheum Dis Clin North Am 1996;22(2):285-303.

(333)   Ahles TA, Yunus MB, Masi AT. Is chronic pain a variant of depressive disease? The case of
        primary fibromyalgia syndrome. Pain 1987;29(1):105-11.

(334)   Ahles TA, Khan SA, Yunus MB et al. Psychiatric status of patients with primary fibromyalgia,
        patients with rheumatoid arthritis, and subjects without pain: a blind comparison of DSM-III
        diagnoses. Am J Psychiatry 1991;148(12):1721-6.

(335)   Alfici S, Sigal M, Landau M. Primary fibromyalgia syndrome--a variant of depressive
        disorder? Psychother Psychosom 1989;51(3):156-61.

(336)   Clark S, Campbell SM, Forehand ME et al. Clinical characteristics of fibrositis. II. A "blinded,"
        controlled study using standard psychological tests. Arthritis Rheum 1985;28(2):132-7.

(337)   Dailey PA, Bishop GD, Russell IJ, Fletcher EM. Psychological stress and the
        fibrositis/fibromyalgia syndrome. J Rheumatol 1990;17(10):1380-5.

(338)   Hawley DJ, Wolfe F. Depression is not more common in rheumatoid arthritis: a 10-year
        longitudinal study of 6,153 patients with rheumatic disease. J Rheumatol 1993;20(12):2025-
        31.

(339)   Hudson JI, Hudson MS, Pliner LF et al. Fibromyalgia and major affective disorder: a
        controlled phenomenology and family history study. Am J Psychiatry 1985;142(4):441-6.

(340)   Kirmayer LJ, Robbins JM, Kapusta MA. Somatization and depression in fibromyalgia
        syndrome. Am J Psychiatry 1988;145(8):950-4.

(341)   Krag NJ, Norregaard J, Larsen JK, Danneskiold-Samsoe B. A blinded, controlled evaluation of anxiety and depressive symptoms in patients with fibromyalgia, as measured by standardized psychometric interview scales. Acta Psychiatr Scand 1994;89(6):370-5.

(342)   Walker EA, Keegan D, Gardner G et al. Psychosocial factors in fibromyalgia compared with rheumatoid arthritis: I. Psychiatric diagnoses and functional disability. Psychosom Med 1997;59(6):565-71.

(343)   Walker EA, Keegan D, Gardner G et al. Psychosocial factors in fibromyalgia compared with rheumatoid arthritis: II. Sexual, physical, and emotional abuse and neglect. Psychosom Med 1997;59(6):572-7.

(344)   Kassam A, Patten SB. Major depression, fibromyalgia and labour force participation: a population-based cross-sectional study. BMC Musculoskelet Disord 2006;7:4.

(345)   White KP, Nielson WR, Harth M et al. Chronic widespread musculoskeletal pain with or without fibromyalgia: psychological distress in a representative community adult sample. J Rheumatol 2002;29(3):588-94.

(346)   Radloff L. The CES-D scale: a self-report depression scale for research in the general population. Appl Psych Meas 1977;1:385-401.

(347)   Speilberger C, Gorsuch RL, Vagg PR, Jacobs GR. The State-Trait Anxiety Inventory. Palo Alto, CA: Consulting Psychologists Press; 1977.

(348)   Sagen U, Vik TG, Moum T et al. Screening for anxiety and depression after stroke: comparison of the hospital anxiety and depression scale and the Montgomery and Asberg depression rating scale. J Psychosom Res 2009;67(4):325-32.

(349)   Irwin M, Clark C, Kennedy B et al. Nocturnal catecholamines and immune function in insomniacs, depressed patients, and control subjects. Brain Behav Immun 2003;17:365-72.

(350)   Jozuka H, Jozuka E, Takeuchi S, Nishikaze O. Comparison of immunological and endocrinological markers associated with major depression. J Int Med Res 2003;31:36-41.

(351)   Maddock C, Pariante CM. How does stress affect you? An overview of stress, immunity, depression and disease. Epidemiol Psychiatr Soc 2001;10:153-62.

(352)   Raison CL, Miller AH. The neuroimmunology of stress and depression. Semin Clin Neuropsychiatry 2001;6:272947.

(353)   Tomassini C, Rosina A, Billari FC et al. The effect of losing the twin and losing the partner on mortality. Twin Res 2002;5:210-7.

(354)   Martikainen P, Valkonen T. Mortality after the death of a spouse: rates and causes of death in a large Finnish cohort. I. Am J Public Health 1996;86:1087-93.

(355)   Smith KR, Zick CD. Risk of mortality following widowhood: age and sex differences by mode of death. Soc Biol 1996;43:59-71.

(356)   Yunus MB. Primary fibromyalgia syndrome: current concepts. Compr Ther 1984;10:21-8.

(357)   Bennett RM. Disabling fibromyalgia: Appearance versus reality. J Rheumatol
        1993;21(11):1821-4.

(358)   Romano TJ. Valid complaints or malingering? Clinical experiences with post-traumatic
        fibromyalgia syndrome. West Virg Med J 1990;86(198).

(359)   Waylonis GW, Perkins RH. Post-traumatic fibromyalgia. Amer J Phys Med Rehab
        1994;73(6):403-12.

(360)   Rush PJ, Ameis A. Trauma and fibromyalgia: Does the punishment fit the crime? [letter]. J
        Rheumatol 1995;22(2):372.

(361)   White KP, Harth M, Speechley M, Ostbye T. Fibromyalgia in Rheumatology Practice: A
        Survey of Canadian Rheumatologists. J Rheumatol 1995;22(4):722-6.

(362)   Marder WD, Meenan RF, Felson DT et al. The Present and Future Adequacy of
        Rheumatology Manpower. Arthritis Rheum, 1991;34:1209-1217 1991;34:1209-17.

(363)   Calabozo-Raluy M, Llamazares-Gonzales AI, Munoz-Gallo MT, Alonso-Ruiz A. Sindrome de
        Fibromialgia (Fibrositis); Tan Frequente Como Desconcido. Med Clin Barc 1990;94:173-5.

(364)   Reilly PA, Littlejohn GO. Peripheral Arthralgic Presentation of Fibrositis/Fibromyalgia
        Syndrome. J Rheumatol 1992;19:281-3.

(365)   Hartz A, Kirchdoerfer E. Undetected fibrositis in primary care practice. J Fam Pract
        1987;25:365-9.

(366)   Forseth KO, Gran JT, Husby G. A population study of the incidence of fibromyalgia among
        females aged 26 - 55 years. Arthritis Rheum 1997;40 (suppl):S44.

(367)   Hawley DJ, Wolfe F. Pain, disability, and pain/disability relationships in seven rheumatic
        disorders: A study of 1,522 patients. J Rheumatol, 1991; 18 (10): 1552-57 1991;18(10):1552-
        7.

(368)   Burckhardt CS, Clark SR, Bennett RM. Fibromyalgia and quality of life: A comparative
        analysis. J Rheumatol 1993;20(3):475-9.

(369)   Callahan LF, Smith WJ, Pincus T. Self-reported questionnaires in five rheumatic diseases.
        Comparisons of health status constructs and associations with formal education level.
        Arthritis Care Res 1989;2:122-31.

(370)   Mengshoel AM, Forre O. Pain and fatigue in patients with rheumatic disorders. Clin
        Rheumatol 1993;12(4):515-21.

(371)   Viitanen JV, Kautiainen H, Isomaki H. Pain intensity in patients with fibromyalgia and
        rheumatoid arthritis. Scand J Rheumatol 1993;22:131-5.

(372)   Gladman DD, Urowitz MB, Gough J, MacKinnon A. Fibromyalgia is a major contributor to quality of life in lupus. J Rheumatol 1997;24(11):2145-8.

(373)   Wolfe F, Anderson J, Harkness D et al. Work and disability status of persons with fibromyalgia. J Rheumatol 1997;24(6):1171-8.

(374)   McCain GA, Cameron R, Kennedy JC. The problem of long term disability payments and litigation in primary fibromyalgia: The Canadian perspective. J Rheumatol 1989;16((suppl 16)):174-6.

(375)   Bengtsson A, Henriksson K-G, Jorfeldt L et al. Primary fibromyalgia. A clinical and laboratory study of 55 patients. Scand J Rheumatol 1986;15:340-7.

(376)   Ledingham J, Doherty S, Doherty M. Primary fibromyalgia syndrome - an outcome study. Br J Rheumatol 1993;32:139-42 1993;32:139-42.

(377)   Bruusgaard D, Evensen AR, Bjerkedal T. Fibromyalgia - A New Cause For Disability Pension. Scand J Soc Med 1993;1993(21):116-9.

(378)   White KP, Speechley M, Harth M, Ostbye T. The London fibromyalgia epidemiology study (LFES): Estimating the number of Canadian adults with fibromyalgia (FMS). Arthritis Rheum 2010;40:S187.

(379)   White KP, Speechley M, Harth M, Ostbye T. The London fibromyalgia epidemiology study: Direct health care costs of fibromyalgia syndrome in London Ontario. J Rheumatol 1999;26:885-9.

(380)   Wolfe F, Anderson J, Harkness D et al. A prospective, longitudinal multicenter study of service utilization and costs in fibromyalgia. Arthritis Rheum 2010;40:1560-70.

(381)   White KP, Harth M. An analytical review of 24 controlled fibromyalgia (FMS) clinical trials. Pain 1996;64(2):211-9.

(382)   Carrette S, Bell MJ, Reynolds WJ et al. Comparison of amitriptyline, cyclobenzaprine, and placebo in the treatment of fibromyalgia. A randomized, double-blind clinical trial. Arthritis Rheum 1994;37(1):32-40.

(383)   Carrette S, McCain GA, Bell DA, Fam AG. Evaluation of amitriptyline in primary fibrositis. A double-blind, placebo-controlled study. Arthritis Rheum 1996;29(5):655-9.

(384)   Clark S, Tindall EA, Bennett RM. A double blind crossover trial of prednisone versus placebo in the treatment of fibrositis. J Rheumatol 1985;12(5):980-3.

(385)   Goldenberg DL, Mayskiy M, Mossey C et al. A randomized, double-blind cross-over trial of fluoxetene and amitriptyline in the treatment of fibromyalgia. Arthritis Rheum 1996;39(11):1852-9.

(386)   Quimby LG, Gratwick GM, Whitney CD, Block SR. A randomized trial of cyclobenzaprine for the treatment of fibromyalgia. J Rheumatol 1989;16((suppl 19)):140-3.

(387)   Russell IJ, Fletcher EM, Michalek JE et al. Treatment of primary fibrositis/fibromyalgia
        syndrome with ibuprofen and alprazolam. A double-blind, placebo-controlled study.
        Arthritis Rheum 1991;34(5):552-60.

(388)   Bennett RM. Fibromyalgia and the disability dilemma: A new era in understanding a
        complex, multidimensional pain syndrome. Arthritis Rheum 1996;39(1627):1634.

(389)   Carrette S. Fibromyalgia, disability and compensation: How should we approach this new
        reality? J Can Rheum Assoc 1993;2:6-7.

(390)   Ferguson DA. "RSI" Putting the epidemic to rest. Med J Austral 1987;147:213-4.

(391)   Hocking B. Epidemiological aspects of "repetitive strain injury" in Telecom Australia. Med J
        Austral 1987;147:218-22.

(392)   Hocking B. "Repetitive strain injury" in Telecom Australia [letter]. Med J Austral
        1989;150:724.

(393)   Littlejohn GO. Repetitive strain syndrome: an Australian experience. J Rheumatol (editorial)
        1986;13:1004-6.

(394)   Littlejohn GO. Fibrositis/fibromyalgia in the workplace. Rheum Dis Clin North Am
        1989;15:45-60.

(395)   Miller MH, Topliss DJ. Chronic upper limb pain syndrome (repetitive strain injury) in the
        Australian workforce: A systematic cross sectional rheumatological study of 229 patients. J
        Rheumatol 1988;15:1705-12.

(396)   White KP, Ostbye T, Harth M et al. Perspectives on post-traumatic fibromyalgia: A random
        survey of Canadian general practitioners, orthopedists, physiatrists and rheumatologists. J
        Rheumatol 2000;27(790):796.

(397)   Smith MD. Relationship of fibromyalgia to site and type of trauma: comment on the articles
        by Buskila et al and Aaron et al. Arthritis Rheum 1998;41:378.

(398)   Neumann L, Zeldets V, Bolotin A, Buskila D. Outcome of posttraumatic fibromyalgia: a 3-year
        follow-up of 78 cases of cervical spine injuries. Semin Arthritis Rheum 2003;32(5):320-5.

(399)   Borchgrevink GE, Lereim I, Royneland L et al. National health insurance consumption and
        chronic symptoms following mild neck sprain injuries in car collisions. Scand J Soc Med
        1996;24:264-71.

(400)   Radanov BP, Sturzenegger M, Di Stefano G. Long-term outcome after whiplash injury: a 2-
        year follow up considering features of injury mechanism and somatic, radiologic, and
        psychosocial findings. Medicine (Baltimore) 1975;74:281-97.

(401)   Harder S, Veilleux M, Suissa S. The effect of socio-demographic and crash-related factors on
        the prognosis of whiplash. J Clin Epidemiol 1998;51:377-84.

(402) Bykund PO, Bjornstig U. Sick leave and disability pension among passenger car occupants injured in urban traffic. Spine 1998;23:1023-8.

(403) Al-Allaf AW, Dunbar KL, Hallum NS et al. A case-control study examining the role of physical trauma in the onset of fibromyalgia syndrome. Rheumatology (Oxford) 2002;41(4):450-3.

(404) Tishler M, Levy O, Maslakov I et al. Neck injury and fibromyalgia-- are they really associated? J Rheumatol 2006;33(6):1183-5.

(405) Obelieniene D, Schrader H, Bovim G et al. Pain after whiplash: a prospective controlled inception cohort study. J Neurol Neurosurg Psychiatry 1999;66(3 279):283.

(406) Obelieniene D, Bovim G, Schrader H et al. Headache after whiplash: a historical cohort study outside the medico-legal context. Cephalalgia 2010;18(8):559-64.

(407) Schrader H, Obelieniene D, Bovim G et al. Natural evolution of late whiplash syndrome outside the medicolegal context. Lancet 1996;347(9010):1207-11.

(408) Buskila D, Neumann L. Musculoskeletal injury as a trigger for fibromyalgia/posttraumatic fibromyalgia. Curr Rheumatol Rep 2000;2(2):104-8.

(409) Saskin P, Moldofsky H, Lue FA. Sleep and post-traumatic pain modulation disorder (fibrositis syndrome). Psychosom Med 1986;48(319):323.

(410) Gupta MA, Moldofsky H. Dysthymic disorder and rheumatic pain disorder (fibrositis syndrome): a comparison of symptoms and sleep physiology. Can J Psychiatry 1986;31:608-16.

(411) Moldofsky H. Sleep and musculoskeletal pain. Am J Med 1986;81((Suppl 3A)):85-9.

(412) Hardy JD, Wott HG, Goodell H. Experimental evidence on the nature of cutaneous hyperalgesia. J Clin Invest 1950;29:115-40.

(413) Aprill C, Dwyer A, Bogduk N. Cervical zygapophyseal joint pain patterns II: A clinical evaluation. Spine 1990;15(6):458-61.

(414) Dwyer A, Aprill C, Bogduk N. Cervical zygapophyseal joint pain patterns I: A study in normal volunteers. Spine 1990;15(6):453-7.

(415) Lord SM, Barnsley L, Wallis BJ et al. Percutaneous radio-frequency neurotomy for chronic cervical zygapophyseal-joint pain. N Engl J Med 1996;335:1721-6.

(416) Wallis BJ, Lord SM, Bogduk N. Resolution of psychological distress of whiplash patients following treatment by radio-frequency neurotomy: a randomized, double-blind, placebo-controlled trial. Pain 1997;73:15-22.

(417) Smythe HA. The 'repetitive strain injury syndrome' is referred pain from the neck. J Rheumatol 1988;15:1604-8.

(418) Smythe HA. The C6-7 syndrome - clinical features and treatment response. J Rheumatol 1994;21:1520-6.

(419) Zimmerman M. Pathophysiological mechanisms of fibromyalgia. Clin J Pain 1991;7((suppl 7)):S8-S15.

(420) Coderre TJ, Katz J, Vaccarino AL, Melzack R. Contribution of central neuroplasticity to pathological pain: review of clinical and experimental evidence. Pain52259285 1993.

(421) Brylin M, Hindfelt B. Ear pain due to myocardial ischaemia. Am Heart J 1984;107(186):187.

(422) Neugebauer V, Schaible HG. Evidence for a central component in the sensitization of spinal neurons with joint input during acute arthritis in cat's knee. J Neurophysiol 1990;64:299-311.

(423) Woolf CJ. Long term alterations in the excitability of the flexion reflex produced by peripheral tissue injury in the chronic decerebrate rat. Pain 1984;18:325-43.

(424) Wall PD, Scadding JW, Tomkiewicz MM. The production and prevention of experimental anesthesia dolorosa. Pain 1979;6:179-82.

(425) Katz J, Vaccarino AL, Coderre TJ, Melzack R. Injury prior to neurectomy alters the pattern of autonomy in rats: behavioural evidence of central neural plasticity. Anesthesiology 1991;75:876-83.

(426) Mense S. Referral of muscle pain. American Pain Society J 1994;3:10-2.

(427) Molander C, Ygge I, Dalsgaard CJ. Substance P, somatostatin- and calcitonin gene-related peptide-like immunoreactivity and fluoride resistant acid phosphatase-activity in relation to retrograde labelled cutaneous, muscular and visceral primary sensory neurons in the rat. Neurosci Lett;74:34-42. Neurosci Lett 1987;74(1):34-42.

(428) Sastry BR. Substance P effects on spinal nociceptive neurons. Life Sci 1979;24:2169-78.

(429) Zieglgansberger W, Tolloch IF. Effects of substance P on neurons in the dorsal horn of the spinal cord of the cat. Brain Res 1979;166:273-82.

(430) Agnati LF, Fuxe K, Zoli M et al. A correlation analysis of the regional distribution of central enkephalin and beta-endorphin immunoreactive terminals and of opiate receptors in adult and old male rats: evidence for the existence of two main types of communication in the central nervous system: the volume transmission and the wiring transmission. Acta Physiol Scand 1986;128:201-7.

(431) Russell IJ. Advances in fibromyalgia: possible role for central neurochemicals. Am J Med Sci 1998;315:377-84.

(432) Bradley LA, Alarcon GS, Sotolongo A et al. Cerebrospinal fluid (CSF) levels of substance P (SP) are abnormal in patients with fibromyalgia (FM) regardless of traumatic or insidious pain onset. Arthritis Rheum 1998;41((suppl)):S256.

(433) Weigent DA, Bradley LA, Blalock JE, Alarcon GS. Current concepts in the pathophysiology of abnormal pain perception in fibromyalgia. Am J Med Sci 1998;315:405-12.

(434) Radanov BP, Sturzenegger M. Predicting recovery from common whiplash. Eur Neurol 1996;36:48-51.

(435) Sturzenegger M, Di Stefano G, Radanov BP, Schnidrig A. Presenting symptoms and signs after whiplash injury: the influence of accident mechanisms. Neurology 1994;44(688):693.

(436) Gargan M, Bannister G, Main C, Hollis S. The behavioural response to whiplash injury. J Bone Joint Surg 1997;79:523-6.

(437) Borchgrevink GE, Stiles TC, Borchgrevink PC, Lereim I. Personality profile among symptomatic and recovered patients with neck sprain injury, measured by MCMI-I acutely and at 6 months after car accidents. J Psychosom Res 1997;42:357-67.

(438) Lanier DC, Stockton P. Clinical predictors of outcome of acute episodes of low back pain. J Family Pract 1988;27:483-9.

(439) Burton AK, Tillotson KM, Main C, Hollis S. Psychosocial predictors of outcome in acute and subchronic low back trouble. Spine 1995;20:722-8.

(440) Von Korff M, Deyo RACD, Barlow W. Back pain in primary care. Outcomes at 1 year. Spine 1993;18:855-62.

(441) Schrader H, Obelieniene D, Bovim G et al. Natural evolution of late whiplash syndrome outside the medicolegal context. Lancet 1996;347(9010):1207-11.

(442) Reilly PA, Travers R, Littlejohn GO. Epidemiology of soft tissue rheumatism: the influence of the law. [editorial]. J Rheumatol 1991;18:1448-9.

(443) Mayou R, Tyndel S, Bryant B. Long-term outcome of motor vehicle accident injury. Psychosom Med 2010;59:578-84.

(444) Pennie B, Agambar L. Patterns of injury and recovery in whiplash. Injury 1991;22:57-9. Injury 1991;22:57-9.

(445) Robinson RL, Birnbaum HG, Morley MA et al. Economic cost and epidemiological characteristics of patients with fibromyalgia claims. J Rheumatol 2003;30(6):1318-25.

(446) Martinez JE, Ferraz MB, Sata EI, Atra E. Fibromyalgia versus rheumatoid arthritis: A longitudinal comparison of the quality of life. J Rheumatol 1995;22(2):270-4.

(447) Robinson DJr, Aguilar D, Schoenwetter M et al. Impact of systemic lupus erythematosus on health, family, and work: the patient perspective. Arthritis Care Res (Hoboken) 2010;62(2):266-73.

(448) Fries JF, Spitz P, Kraines RG, Holman HR. Measurement of patient outcome in arthritis. Arthritis Rheum 1980;23(2):137-45.

(449)   Health Assessment Questionnaire Disability Index. Stanford University 2003;Available from: URL: http://aramis.stanford.edu/downloads/HAQ%20-%20DI%202007.pdf

(450)   Meenan RF, Gertman PM, Mason JH. Measuring health status in arthritis. The arthritis impact measurement scales. Arthritis Rheum 1980;23(2):146-52.

(451)   Meenan RF, Gertman PM, Mason JH, Dunaif R. The arthritis impact measurement scales. Further investigations of a health status measure. Arthritis Rheum 1982;25(9):1048-53.

(452)   Health Assessment Questionnaire Disability Index. Stanford University 2003;Available from: URL: http://aramis.stanford.edu/downloads/HAQ%20-%20DI%202007.pdf

(453)   Burckhardt CS, Clark SR, Bennett RM. The fibromyalgia impact questionnaire: Development and validation. J Rheum 1991;18:728-33.

(454)   The Fibromyalgia Impact Questionnaire. DrLowe com 2010;Available from: URL: http://www.drlowe.com/clincare/clinicalforms/fiq.pdf

(455)   Waddell G, McCulloch J, Kummel E, Venner R. Nonorganic Physical Signs in Low-Back Pain. Spine 1980;5(2):117-25.

(456)   Main C, Waddell G. Behavioral Responses to Examination: A Reappraisal of the Interpretation of 'Nonorganic Signs'. Spine 1998;23(21):2367-71.

(457)   Fishbain D, Cole B, Cutler RB et al. A Structured Evidence-Based Review on the Meaning of Nonorganic Physical Signs: Waddell Signs. Pain Medicine (American Academy of Pain Medicine) 2003;4(2):141-81.

(458)   Fishbain D, Cutler RB, Steele Rosomoff R. Is There a Relationship Between Nonorganic Physical Findings (Waddell Signs) and Secondary Gain/Malingering? Clinical Journal of Pain (American Academy of Pain Medicine) 2004;20(6):399-408.

(459)   Calkins DR, Rubenstein LV, Cleary PD et al. Failure of physicians to recognize functional disability in ambulatory patients. Ann Intern Med 1991;114(6):451-454.

(460)   Yelin EH, Henke CJ, Epstein WV. Work disability among persons with musculoskeletal conditions. Arthritis Rheum 1986;29(11):1322-33.

(461)   Liang MH, Daltroy LH, Larson MG et al. Evaluation of Social Security disability in claimants with rheumatic disease. Ann Intern Med 1991;115(1):26-31.

(462)   Simms RW, Roy SH, Hrovat M et al. Lack of association between fibromyalgia syndrome and abnormalities in muscle energy metabolism. Arthritis Rheum 1994;37:794-800.

(463)   Kuchinad A, Schweinhardt P, Seminowicz DA et al. Accelerated brain gray matter loss in fibromyalgia patients: premature aging of the brain? J Neurosci 2007;27(15):4004-7.

(464)   Staud R. Evidence of involvement of central neural mechanisms in generating fibromyalgia pain. Curr Rheumatol Rep 2002;4(4):299-305.

(465)   Staud R, Smitherman ML. Peripheral and central sensitization in fibromyalgia: pathogenetic role. Curr Pain Headache Rep 2002;6(4):259-66.

(466)   Stevens A, Batra A, Kötter I et al. Both pain and EEG response to cold pressor stimulation occurs faster in fibromyalgia patients than in control subjects. Psychiatry Res 2000;97(2-3):237-47.

(467)   Williams DA, Gracely RH. Biology and therapy of fibromyalgia. Functional magnetic resonance imaging findings in fibromyalgia. Arthritis Res Ther 2006;8(6):224.

(468)   Wood PB, Patterson JC, Sunderland JJ et al. Reduced presynaptic dopamine activity in fibromyalgia syndrome demonstrated with positron emission tomography: a pilot study. J Pain 2007;8(1):51-8.

(469)   Yoldas T, Ozgocmen S, Yildizhan H et al. Auditory p300 event-related potentials in fibromyalgia patients. Yonsei Med J 2003;44(1):89-93.

(470)   Yunus M, Young CS, Saeed SA et al. Positron emission tomography in patients with fibromyalgia syndrome and healthy controls. Arthritis Rheum 2004;51(4):513-8.

(471)   Moldofsky H. Chronobiological influences on fibromyalgia syndrome: theoretical and therapeutic implications. Baillieres Clin Rheumatol 1994;8(4):801-10.

(472)   Crofford LJ. Neuroendocrine abnormalities in fibromyalgia and related disorders. Am J Med Sci 1998;315(6):359-66.

(473)   Russell IJ, Vipraio GA, Morgan WW, Bowden CL. Is there a metabolic basis for the fibrositis syndrome? Am J Med 1986;81(3A):50-4.

(474)   Staud R, Domingo M. Evidence for abnormal pain processing in fibromyalgia syndrome. Pain Med 2001;2(3):208-15.

(475)   Staud R, Price DD, Robinson ME et al. Maintenance of windup of second pain requires less frequent stimulation in fibromyalgia patients compared to normal controls. Pain 2004;110(3):689-96.

(476)   White KP, Nielson WR. Cognitive behavioral treatment of fibromyalgia syndrome: a followup assessment. J Rheumatol 1995;22(4):717-21.

(477)   Clifford JC. Successful management of chronic pain syndrome. Can Fam Physician 1993;39:549-59.

(478)   Catchlove R, Cohen K. Effects of a directive return to work approach in the treatment of workman's compensation patients with chronic pain. Pain 1982;14(2):181-91.

(479)   Mayer TG, Gatchel RJ, Mayer H et al. A prospective two-year study of functional restoration in industrial low back injury. An objective assessment procedure. JAMA 1987;258(13):1763-7.

(480) Hazard RG, Fenwick JW, Kalisch SM et al. Functional restoration with behavioral support. A one-year prospective study of patients with chronic low-back pain. Spine (Philadelphia, Pa 1976) 1989;14(2):157-61.

(481) Yunus MB. Fibromyalgia syndrome and myofascial pain syndrome: clinical features, laboratory tests, diagnosis, and pathophysiologic mechanisms. In: Rachlin ES, editor. Myofascial Pain and Fibromyalgia: Trigger Point Management. St. Louis, MO: Mosby-Year Book, Inc.; 1994.

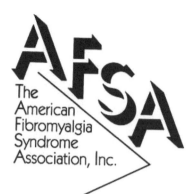

Help Us Fund Fibromyalgia Research

The American Fibromyalgia Syndrome Association (AFSA) is the nation's leading 501(c)3 nonprofit organization dedicated to funding promising new research that accelerates the pace of medical discoveries to improve the quality of life for patients with fibromyalgia.

More than 90% of your donations go to support our mission. Funding research since 1994.

Donate online at **www.afsafund.org**, call **(520) 733-1570**, or clip and send us your contribution below:

Name: _____

Address: _____

City:_____ State: _____

Zip:_____ Country:_____

Phone : (_____) _____

E-mail: _____

❑ Check/MO enclosed   ❑ MasterCard   ❑ VISA

Card Number:_____

Expiration Date:_____

Authorized Signature:_____
* Donations outside the U.S. can only be made online or with a credit card.

AFSA • PO Box 32698 • Tucson, AZ 85751 • USA

Your Contributions
Make A Difference

The American Fibromyalgia Syndrome Association (AFSA) is solely supported by generous donations from patients and their families. As an independent organization, AFSA is not supported by pharmaceutical companies or advertisements. Projects with the greatest promise to benefit patients are selected without third-party influence. We invite you to tell us what types of projects or areas of study you feel should be funded.

People with fibromyalgia deserve:

- ♦ treatments that work
- ♦ blood tests that help guide therapies and measure their effectiveness
- ♦ bodies that can function on a reliable basis
- ♦ to be viewed as having a credible disease

All four of the above goals are of equal importance for improving the quality of life for millions of fibromyalgia patients.

Contribution Categories *(in U.S. funds)*

❑ Friends $25
❑ Inspirations $50
❑ Motivators $100
❑ Visionaries . . . $500
❑ Champions . . . $1,000
❑ Heros . . . $10,000 +
❑ Any size donation
  is welcome! $_____

If you would like to make an "In Memory of" donation, please use a separate sheet of paper to tell us who you would like to memorialize and who we should notify of the donation.

❑ *Check here if you would like your donation to be anonymous.*

Total: $ _____

AFSA • PO Box 32698 • Tucson, AZ 85751 • USA
Website: **www.afsafund.org**
Phone: **(520) 733-1570** • Fax: **(520) 290-5550**

Thank you for your support!

Other books by Dr. Kevin White

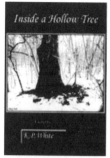

Inside a Hollow Tree (novel, coming January 2011)
K. P. White
$14.95
www.wortleyroadbooks.com

Dalton Hobby was no ordinary boy. With 14 years of abuse and neglect in his past, he now heads off to boarding school, carrying with him nothing but a small suitcase and a green garbage bag full of secrets. But, as each secret is revealed, everyone learns what an extraordinary boy he is.

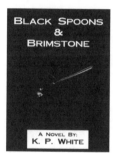

Black Spoons & Brimstone (novel, coming spring 2011)
K. P. White
$14.95
www.wortleyroadbooks.com

Julian Briscoe knew that this was going to be a very, very bad day. One — he had woken up, all alone, in a smelly, horrible place in the middle of nowhere. Two — he had woken up dead.

Other books by Wortley Road Books

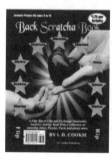

The Back Scratcha Book (child-guardian activity book)
I. D. Cookie (a.k.a. Darlene Steele)
$34.95
www.wortleyroadbooks.com

A flip, rip or clip and exchange interactive surprise activity book with a collection of amusing jokes, puzzles, facts and plenty more. PERFECT for the parent, grandparent or other child guardian who wants to spend quality quiet time with a child between the ages of 9 and 13.

Breaking Thru the

Fibro Fog

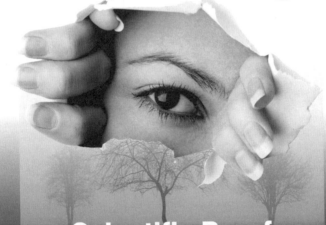

Scientific Proof
Fibromyalgia is Real

Kevin P. White, MD, PhD

Foreword by I. Jon Russell, MD, PhD

``A MUST-READ for ANYONE
with a serious interest in Fibromyalgia``
Tamara K. Liller
President & Director of Publications,
National Fibromyalgia Partnership Inc